KATHY SMITH'S

GETTING BETTER ALL THE TIME

SHAPE UP, EAT SMART, FEEL GREAT!

WARNER BOOKS

A Time Warner Company

ALSO BY KATHY SMITH

Kathy Smith's WalkFit for a Better Body
Kathy Smith's Fitness Makeover

Published by Warner Books, Inc.

PUBLISHER'S NOTE: Neither this nor any other diet or exercise program should be followed without first consulting a health care professional. If you have any special conditions requiring attention, you should consult with your health care professional regularly regarding possible modification of the program contained in this book.

Grateful acknowledgment is given to *Shape* magazine for permission to use the August 1984 and April 1995 covers.

Copyright © 1998 by Kathy Smith Enterprises, Inc.
All rights reserved.

Warner Books, Inc., 1271 Avenue of the Americas, New York, NY 10020
Visit our Web site at http://warnerbooks.com

 A Time Warner Company

Printed in the United States of America
First Printing: February 1998
10 9 8 7 6 5 4 3 2 1

Library of Congress Cataloging-in-Publication Data

Smith, Kathy.
    [Getting better all the time]
    Kathy Smith's getting better all the time : shape up, eat smart,
feel great! / Kathy Smith.
        p. cm.
    Includes index.
    ISBN 0-446-51848-4
    1. Physical fitness for women. 2. Exercise for women. 3. Women—
Health and hygiene. I. Title.
RA781.S6133 1998
613.7'045—dc21   97-26083
                                                                CIP

Book design and composition by L&G McRee
Exercise photos by Ted & Debbie

Acknowledgments

I would like to take a moment to thank several people who helped me with this project. First, Cathy Harris who helped launch this book. Her ability to listen to me and organize my thoughts brought the first focus to the theme of the powerful choices we have in our lives.

Joel Engel brought exceptional writing skills to the project. He kept us focused, on deadline, and offered great insights into the organization and presentation of this material. Beyond that, Joel believed in my message. He is a great coach, a terrific writer, and now, a good friend.

Bonnie Modugno, M.S., R.D., collaborated on the nutrition portion of this book, but her input can be felt throughout. She is a woman of integrity who has tremendous respect for all those people who struggle with diets. Bonnie threw herself into all aspects of this project and for that I'll always be grateful.

Candice Copeland, as usual, has been a true friend and dedicated consultant on the exercise portion of the book. With her husband, Douglas Brooks, she has always been willing to brainstorm ideas, and bring the message of fitness to the public.

Russ Kamalski is my hero. During the highs and lows of this project he kept our team together. On top of that, I would need an entire book to talk about how Russ helps every part of my business. He's always there to keep me going—from the smallest detail, to the big picture, Russ rules!

To the office staff, Gina Marie Soto and Erin Toth. Thanks for your long nights on the computer, at the copier, and on the phones doing research. To Linda Shelton for knowing when to tuck—to Steven Radiloff, for his inspiration and mediation—and to Laurine DiRocco my friend and confidante, thanks to you all.

Finally, to my husband, Steve, for his tireless support and his courage to make powerful choices in his life. And to the two daughters who bring me so much joy, Kate and Perrie. You are too loving for words.

Contents

Contents

Introduction

The fact that you picked up this book probably means that somewhere inside of you is a voice, either whispering or shouting that you're fed up with being overweight, or tired, or bored, and you want someone or something to help you. That's exactly what I'd like to do. My purpose in writing this book is to share with you the important role that the power of choice has made throughout my life. I want you to begin making positive choices, the kind that will help you get the best out of your own life. You do that by making choices that make you more healthy and physically fit.

Just desiring health or wishing you could be fit won't get you there. Actually achieving it requires tapping into the power of choice—that is, choosing a healthier, more physically fit lifestyle. And you can do that by following this book's simple step-by-step program to a better life: The Power of Choice Plan.

This is a book about choices. The choices that we all have the ability to make if we want our lives to be better. Specifically, choosing to be healthier and happier, more fit, and more self-satisfied. These are the most profound choices you'll ever make, because they have the power to change everything else in your life, including personal relationships.

We all make choices every day: *Now or later? Here or there? Him or her? This or that? Should I or shouldn't I?*

In fact, you could reasonably say that life is an endless series of choices. They confront us every waking minute. *Watch TV or read the paper? Exercise before work or sleep in? Hot fudge sundae or fresh raspberries?*

Even when we're unaware of the choices or don't recognize them as such, they're still there to be made—and we're still making them.

And while it's true that we may not choose our circumstances at any given moment, we do absolutely choose our reaction to those circumstances. We can put the best face on our situation or the worst. We can look on the bright side or on the dark side. We can start doing something today—learning a new skill, for example— that just may turn tomorrow into a more wonderful and fulfilling day than today. In our daily struggle for self-satisfaction and contentment, choice is our most powerful weapon. Every day, choices supply us with the power to make our lives better.

Yes, knowing that we possess that power can be upsetting and confusing. We often get emotional when presented with choices. The more choices, the more confused we may become—to the point that we sometimes shut down or ignore our options. What happens is that we subconsciously fear upsetting the status quo: No matter how bad things seem now, at least they're familiar. It's that old story of not wanting to change the life you have, no matter how unsatisfying, for the terror of the unknown. But what you miss sometimes is a better life.

This book will focus on those choices that lead to better fitness and health, which also lead to a better quality of life. Think of it as your personal spring cleaning. You know how it is. All you started out to do was straighten up your closet, but you figure, *Well, as long as I'm doing this, I can't very well leave that alone.* With one mess cleaned up, that still untidy pile next to it can no longer be ignored. So one thing leads to another, leads to another, leads to another. In the same way, improving one part of your life will start a domino effect that eventually touches every other aspect of your life making your overall life better.

Health comes along, usually accompanied by other blessings, when you choose to embrace it—which means that you make it a priority. Which means reexamining your current priorities and, if necessary, reordering them. By adopting a healthier lifestyle, one that accommodates exercise, better eating habits, and a new attitude, success will follow.

You might think the only measure of success is money, cars, the latest fashions, or your job description. I disagree. I think that it's up to each of us to define the concept for ourselves.

I recently heard Secretary of State Madeleine Albright describe

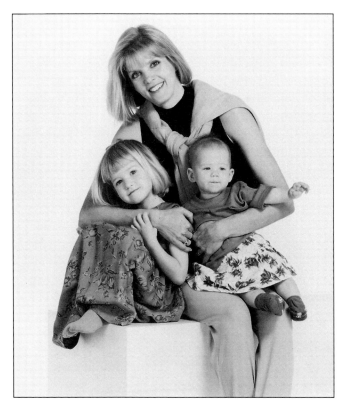

Katie and Perrie always remind me of what's important in life.

success as discovering what it is you love doing, and finding a way to make that your life's work. I suppose Secretary Albright's definition applies to me as well. Long before there was such a thing as the "fitness industry," I knew only that running, exercising, and learning about how and why they affected the human body gave me intense pleasure. It never occurred to me twenty-five years ago that I could make a living doing what I loved. But I'm not a success just because I happen to occupy a corner of the fitness industry. No, I'm a success in my own heart because I am constantly working toward creating a happy balance between work and home. I am always looking for ways to better my life and to help others better theirs. After all, striving to "Get Better All the Time" is exactly what my life is about.

You see, each of us is the sum of the choices we've made up to this point in our lives. What you see when you look at yourself and your surroundings represents choices you began making years ago. And, since you're still making them today, you are continually shaping your destiny. The path you decide to take does not have a destination. It is a road that's always under construction, and the course can be changed whenever you decide.

My sincerest hope is that reading this book will help you learn to recognize how those choices contributed to who you are and, conversely, give you powerful information you need and the motivation it takes to make the necessary changes for you to obtain a better life. Your life is a constant journey toward getting better and I'd like to help you along on this journey by showing you how making better health and fitness choices can improve your body and state of mind.

You begin this process by simply realizing that your life is indeed a succession of choices, and that it's never too late to begin choosing wisely. As the saying goes, "Today is the first day of the rest of your life." As familiar as these words may sound, they are as true as any uttered.

I want you to have a great life, a life you'll love living. My Power of Choice Plan will help you to achieve this. The Plan is broken down into three parts. In Part One, The Power of Miracles, you will learn how to create your own miracle, to make changes that will create a better life for you. I will introduce you to the seven keys to success that I've observed in people who have created their own miracles, and made their dreams come true. I will teach you how to incorporate these steps into your life in order to make it better.

In Part Two, The Power of Food, you'll learn to make your own healthy decisions about food. I'll show you how to become a "functional" eater, someone who understands their needs, and is able to choose the foods that will help to meet those needs. You'll learn how to stop your cravings and lose weight eating the foods you enjoy.

I'll introduce you to three unique meal plans. They all use the same foods, but have subtly distinct and different ratios of carbohydrates, protein, and fat. Though these differences may seem minor to you, they actually have a significant impact on the way your body responds to food. These three plans, "The Starter Plan," "The Carbo Loader," and "The Hunter-Gatherer" were created to help you make better food choices based on your own unique metabolism.

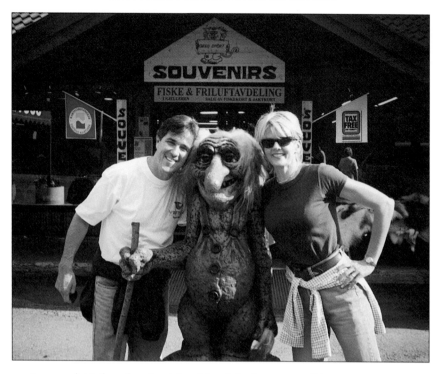

Steve and I take a break with a friend during our walking trip to Norway.

As you determine which food plan works best for you, I want to introduce you to a way of incorporating it into your life so that it becomes a lifestyle. I want you to enjoy as much choice and flexibility with your food as you want or need in order to be consistent. I truly believe that my food program will be a great guide for you as you move toward more functional eating.

My goal is for you to make better food choices, and to become a more independent eater. I've included thirty meal plans and some wonderful recipes for those meal plans that are provided as a foundation for making your own decisions about food. Some of you will want or need more structure to feel "safe," so I'll provide you with the direction and support you need. Others will find yourselves rebelling anytime any food plan feels too constraining. So I'll give you the tools you need to understand your eating so that you can make food choices on your own. This approach is unique in that it teaches you how to work with your body instead of forcing you to eat certain foods.

I will also help you to assess your food behavior by showing you the five levels of eating that we all experience at one time or another. These levels range from dysfunctional eating to optimal eating. I will guide you through these levels and help you to move toward a lifestyle in which you are in control and comfortable with your food choices at all times.

Part Three, The Power of Fitness, focuses on the three key areas of exercise, which are cardiovascular, or "aerobic" exercise, strength training, and flexibility. For aerobics I've designed an all-inclusive Lean Walk System that incorporates intervals, or short energy sprints. It will turn your ordinary walk into a workout while preventing boredom, and it's one of the best ways to train your body to burn calories. The weight training program teaches you how to strengthen and tone your muscles so you can slow down the aging process, boost your metabolism, and lose weight. Finally, the flexibility program focuses on exercise that will keep you limber and reduce stress.

But what I think is the most unusual and important aspect of this program is a concept called "Periodization"—it is a method that will help you vary the type of workout you do, and its intensity. Periodization helps to prevent your body from plateauing, so your progress won't slow down. I will provide you with a six-week plan that will take you week by week through a program that maintains your progress and won't allow you to become bored, or to abandon it.

My hope is that this book will inspire you to discover for yourself how even simple choices can improve your life—its circumstances as well as its quality. I know it's possible because so many thousands of you have written to me or approached me in person over the years to express your thanks for my having contributed to your lives. I assure you, the feeling is absolutely mutual; I appreciate every letter. So in that spirit, let us together take our relationship a few steps farther . . . by beginning **The Power of Choice Plan!**

The Power of Choice

Life is what you make of it.

You've heard that adage a thousand times. But what do the words really mean?

People usually recite them as a means of consolation, when bad things happen to them. They're hoping to persuade you that how you interpret your present circumstances, whether to smile or stay miserable, is up to you.

While that's true enough, I have an additional interpretation. I think you make your life. Period. I'm convinced that you cannot only put the best face on your circumstances but, more important-ly, put yourself in better circumstances—those that are less likely to require a best face.

Look around you. Where you are right now is the destination that represents every step you've ever taken, every road you've ever traveled down, every choice you've ever made. Whatever those choices were, however small or large they seemed at the time—which book to read, whom to date, what shoes to wear—they're all pieces of the jigsaw puzzle that form a picture of you today. Just as turning left on Elm will land you somewhere different from going right, so, too, would you be different if you'd made different choic-es. Each one, in its own way, contributed something to making your life what it is today.

If you like your life, congratulations; you've chosen well. If you don't like what you see when you look around, don't despair. As long as you're alive, you have choices available to you, which means if you're not satisfied with your life, you can always make it better. It's time to begin making better choices, ones that lead to somewhere you want to be. Remember, life is about Getting Better All the Time.

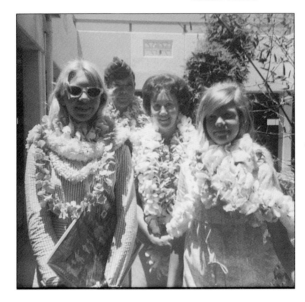

Dad was transferred to Hawaii. Another move for our family; this time no one was complaining.

I was born into a military family, the daughter of an air force pilot whose rise through the ranks required that he relocate every few years. Just when my sister and I would have begun to make friends, we'd be forced to pick up stakes and move somewhere else—Texas, Wisconsin, Brazil, Alabama, Hawaii, Oklahoma, California. As a "professional" military wife, Mom would do her best to adapt to each new location, while Sharon and I tried to learn the styles and attitudes of a new town. It was tough—probably tougher than my rose-colored memories of those times—but we got through because the one constant from place to place was our family's closeness. Dad and I became particularly attached to each other. For security, I relied on his love, his knowledge, his wisdom, his strength, his kindness.

And then he died. Just like that. Heart attack at age forty-two. When I was seventeen.

Dad's death devastated me. But Mom's, two years later in a plane crash, hit even harder. Suddenly I had no idea what would become of me or where I would end up. Suddenly there was no one to rely on, no one to go to for advice, for consolation, for hugs. At a time in my life when I could have used some good parenting, I had to parent myself.

Reaching out to my sister, I expected she'd do the same, while each of us responded to the difficult times. That seemed so logical, felt so right.

A couple of years older than I, Sharon was pretty, smart, and had all the potential I had. But Sharon wasn't there for me. She began reacting to the hand that life had dealt us by focusing on what she'd lost rather than the opportunities ahead. By staying out all night—drinking and taking drugs—she chose not to look toward the future, but rather to dwell on our devastated past.

I chose a path that eventually led to a life of purpose and calling. My sister chose a path of self-destruction that led to some scary places such as alcoholism and drug addiction. Her choices impacted her health, looks, confidence, and self-esteem.

Visiting my sister, Sharon, in Hawaii.

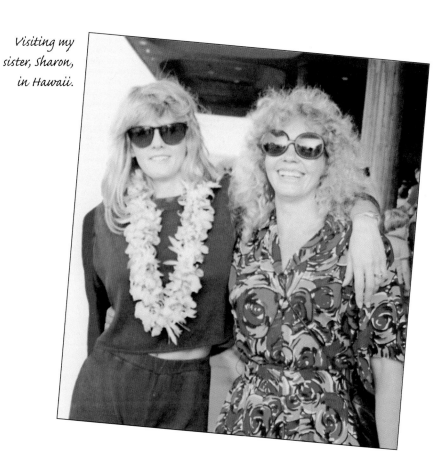

If you don't like what you see when you look around, then it's time for a change. Whether you're overweight, unhappy, or simply bored by life itself, you can become the person you once imagined yourself to be. The way my sister Sharon did. After years of alcoholism and drug addiction, she made one of the most powerful choices anyone can make—she sought help for her addictions. That decision completely changed her life around, to the point where today she's recovered and living a healthy, productive life. And I couldn't be more proud of her.

And therein lie the story and message I want to pass along to you: Your choices today determine your tomorrow and you make your life through the power of choice.

My Turning Point

If I were to tell you that you had to live without air for the rest of your life, you'd know that the rest of your life would last only another minute or so.

If I were to demand that you go forever without water, you'd realize very quickly that "forever" is only a few days more.

And if I ordered you to stop eating food, you'd understand that your life could last only another two painful months.

But if I suggested that you never again exercise, you might be relieved, maybe even ecstatic, to know that you wouldn't ever have to go for a jog, or swim laps, or lift weights.

To me, that's just as crazy as trying to go without air, water, or food—and I think I can persuade you to believe the same. Exercise is probably as important to my well-being as any of those. Which is exactly the way I'd like you to begin thinking. I could no more easily imagine living without regular exercise than without dinner. In some ways, in fact, exercise is actually more critical to my mental and spiritual health than dinner is. While having a plate of pasta or a piece of grilled fish will no doubt hit the spot, no amount of food can ever change my mood the way a good workout can.

I remember when I was living in Hawaii in the 1970s, just after Mom was killed. An emotional basket case, I naturally turned for comfort to my boyfriend Rob, a big, rugged University of Hawaii football player. Well, Rob wasn't exactly equipped to deal with my grief and confusion, so he began pulling away from me—into the arms of other women. At the time, I regarded this as the loss of someone else I loved, the third in a continuing series—Mom, Dad, and now Rob. In awful pain and wondering whether everyone I cared deeply for would either leave me or die, I thought long and hard about my life: What, if anything, was its purpose? Why was I here? Why is this happening to me?

As it turned out, the answers were delivered in a most unusual way. And I have Rob to thank for them. Because of his abandonment, I changed my life.

As an athlete who needed to stay in top physical condition, Rob would go on long runs across the lush landscapes of Oahu. Just to be near him more often, I'd begun running, too. At first I'd been unable to keep up, but then my natural competitive spirit emerged—and with it, my endurance. I know I surprised him with how quickly I progressed, running stride for stride with him mile after mile.

Before long I'd found myself lacing up my sneakers for a run whether or not Rob was going. I began turning more and more to the one activity in my life that gave me confidence, strength, and peace of mind.

Running.

In essence, running became my emotional crutch. Returning from a four- or five-mile jaunt, I'd actually feel as though I'd undergone a cathartic, healing experience. Those endorphins—the brain's natural opiates that are released after exercise—really worked their magic on my state of mind. I found myself able to think more clearly and evaluate my situation with greater objectivity, as opposed to the all-encompassing despair that can infect every thought and feeling with a sense of hopelessness. Yes, I became more hopeful about the future, and my place in it.

Running also became a sort of teacher to me by tuning me into the unheeded messages my body had been sending. Before I began running, the alcohol and drugs I experimented with seemed otherwise harmless. (This was, after all, the 1960s, the era of Vietnam and "Flower Children," when the use of alcohol and recreational drugs was almost a universal rite of passage.) In my body, there were no obvious negative symptoms—until I'd achieved a certain level of fitness. Then I began operating on a higher level and could literally feel these poisons contaminating me.

Not surprisingly, it was during those hour-long runs that I began to evaluate my life with a clear eye toward change. The run itself took on some kind of symbolic significance: Looking ahead on the road I thought about myself and where I'd be in five, ten, fifteen years from now if I continued with my unhealthy lifestyle and destructive relationship. I realized I had the ability to make my life better. And I resolved to do so.

My determination was bolstered by a chance meeting. While running one day, I happened upon a park and saw an incredibly vital man leading exercises for a few middle-aged people. From my spot just within earshot, it seemed obvious to me how animated and full of life this swimsuit-clad man was. So when he announced to his "students" during a break that he was in fact pushing eighty, I had to suppress a shriek. He was nearly twice the age of my father at the time of Dad's death. I couldn't help thinking "what if?"—what if Dad had realized the necessity of staying fit, too? And Mom—this man was twice her age at the time of her death. Even though she'd died in an accident, I had no doubt that she wouldn't have lived to see eighty either, not the way she ate, drank, and smoked.

Later, getting to know this extraordinary man, Paul Bragg, I witnessed up close for myself how a healthy lifestyle impacts every corner of your life.

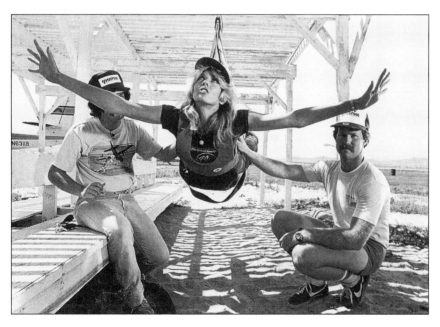

Always up for an adventure! Practicing for my first skydiving experience during my days on Alive & Well. (Yes, my chute opened.)

A healthy lifestyle is the equivalent of getting your car tuned and changing its oil regularly. Of course it's going to drive better, be more responsive, and last longer than one that's neglected. Ask yourself which you'd rather have, a finely tuned precision machine or a coughing, sputtering clunker. When I asked myself that question, I came to the obvious conclusion—the one I hope you, too, arrive at.

Through running, I turned on to other forms of exercise, such as swimming, tennis, weights, rowing, and calisthenics. This was in the era before the so-called fitness industry existed, so a woman doing some of these things raised a few eyebrows. But I didn't care. Everything about exercise excited me. Not only doing it, but also studying it in college classes and through reading. Wherever I had to go to find information, whatever the source, I hungrily devoured anything that contained even a nugget of information about the physiologic processes of exercise, as well as its effects, both mentally and emotionally. I studied biomechanics and kinesiology, nutrition and physiology. I used myself as a laboratory and guinea pig, attacking my experiments with all the passionate glee of a mad scientist certain that she's on the brink of a world-shaking discovery. In fact, I was. Though I took what was at the time "the road less traveled," I did indeed discover that choosing a healthy lifestyle has made all the difference.

It's been nearly twenty-five years since I began walking down that road—a quarter-century of study and participation. And from where I stand now, I can assure you that if some form of regular exercise isn't as important to you as air, water, and food, then you may as well believe that the Earth is flat.

It's time to begin making better choices. Choosing a healthy lifestyle is the most important thing you'll ever do, because whatever else it is that you aim to do in life, being healthy will help you accomplish it. I promise you, adopting a healthy lifestyle isn't going to be as distasteful as having to finish all your Brussels sprouts when you were a kid. It's going to be fun, and, best of all, it's going to change the way you view the world.

For me, running set in motion a process that began with feeling powerless and ended with feeling powerful enough to first trust, then follow, my own instincts. Running helped me to make a life-changing discovery.

This is what I discovered: By picking a physical activity I enjoyed and that challenged me, I derived the confidence and strength from the completion of each day's activity. Little by little I built stamina, and the release of endorphins and the oxygenation of my blood started paying off.

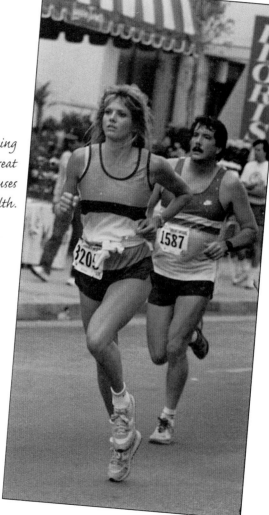

I enjoy running and walking in charity events. It's a great way to contribute to causes and my own health.

I began to feel better. So I began eating healthier. My body insisted on it. I looked better and everyone noticed, because it was obvious. Even to me. I had accomplished something. And I was proud. This then became the building block that laid the foundation for all my goals.

Whenever it seems that my life is out of control, I'll always have this one spot to which I can return, reminding me that I'm the one in charge.

That's how I choose to look at it. And by the time we're through here, so will you! More importantly, you'll have the tools to make the choices you know are in your best interest.

Taking Stock of Your Life

A few months ago, while stopped at a red light not far from my home, I couldn't help reading a billboard hovering above me. The message on it, written in bold, black letters, seemed shocking even for Los Angeles: TOPLESS DRIVING SCHOOL. I knew that there were comedy driving schools, where the instructors were stand-up comics, and driving schools where you got pizza at the end of the eight-hour class. But topless driving schools? "Beautiful female instructors," the sign read, "with unbelievable bodies." I couldn't decide whether I was amused or disgusted.

Only in L.A., I thought. Then I read the fine print at the bottom of the billboard: "This has been a reality check, brought to you by *Buzz* magazine." Obviously, the whole thing was a joke, a stab at irony, intended to test the Los Angeleno's sense of limits. I like to think that, sooner or later, I would have realized it was a joke, even without the disclaimer. But apparently a good many people took the message seriously, because the telephone lines at the Department of Motor Vehicles were jammed with calls from men eager to sign up for the school. So many callers, in fact, that pretty soon *Buzz* was ordered to take down the billboard.

I don't know if any good came of the campaign for anyone else. As for me, I took it as a powerful reminder that we human beings need periodic—make that regular—reality checks. Though not necessarily in the way the billboard intended.

For me, a reality check means taking stock of yourself and your circumstances. For example, when you look in the mirror, do you like whom and what you see? If that's hard, try projecting outward another five, ten, fifteen, twenty-five years. Imagine yourself in those future years. Imagine yourself after another decade or two of doing what you're doing now. How are you going to look? How much are you going to weigh? Where will you be living, and with whom? What will you be doing?

If your projections don't meet your expectations, then you've got work to do. It's time to change your lifestyle for the better, trade in the one you have for one that will support the person you expect and hope to be.

Nathaniel Branden is a philosopher and writer who leads seminars on self-esteem with his wife, Devers. In one workshop I attended, Nathaniel had all of us participate in an exercise that I found extremely powerful. We had to draw, across a sheet of paper, a straight horizontal line with short vertical brackets closing off both the left and right sides. The line, he said, represented each of our lives, with the brackets indicating the times of our birth and eventual death.

After we had a moment to contemplate the power of seeing our lives reduced to a mere symbol, we were told to mark a point anywhere on the line that would indicate where in our lives we thought we were at that moment. The far left point indicated birth, the far right, death. I, like most people, drew my mark about a third of the way from the left. But as Nathaniel pointed out, if you're in your forties—which I and the majority of others were—then the line for the present ought to be more than halfway to the right. With average life expectancies running into the seventies, a forty-year-old is statistically past the halfway mark. I would have to live to the ripe old age of ninety in order to now be at only the halfway mark.

That, to me, was a real wake-up call. A reality check. The question it forced me to answer was, "How do I want to spend the next forty-five years of my life?"

Now think about your life and ask yourself the same question—where are you on the life time line right now?

YOUR LIFE TIME LINE

I--I

BIRTH   DEATH

Your answer is crucially important, and may cause you to reassess how you're living today. Because typically, the final years of life are less vigorous than the younger years. So in those final years, do you want to be confined to a retirement home with somebody caring for your needs, bodily and otherwise? Or do you want to be independent, living every moment to the fullest, playing with your grandchildren, maybe traveling around the world, doing activities you enjoy?

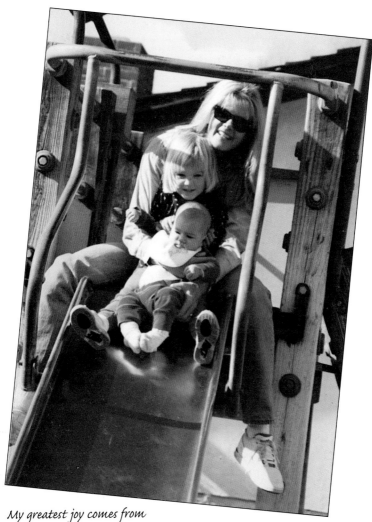

*My greatest joy comes from
spending time with the girls.*

There may not be a more important question for you to answer honestly, with as much precision as you can. It goes to the way you view the world, yourself, and your place in it. It defines your expectations.

I have high expectations and I expect that when I get to be an old woman I'll still be skiing, playing tennis, running 10-Ks, traveling, and still learning. I expect I'll be down on the floor with my grandkids, rolling around and giggling, being even sillier than they are. I can imagine doing these things, as opposed to wishing what might have been.

The reason I expect so much of the future is that I intend to maintain my health and fitness. Quality of life, even more than the quantity, is what I'm after. I want to be active and involved. Dying doesn't scare me. Not being able to enjoy life when I'm alive does.

In a way, my parents' early death taught me, at a young age, to cherish the gift of life we've been given, not to take it for granted, and not to waste it. Fitness allows you to appreciate what life has to offer—that is, not be held back by an aching this or a sore that.

Fit now, fit forever. That's my motto.

The notion that most of us carry around in our head, that we're not going to die, is a destructive one. As we rush from one chore to the next—getting the kids off to school, grocery shopping, working all day, etc.—it not only keeps us from taking better care of ourselves in the present, it also sabotages our instinct to "stop and smell the roses" along our path. In my experience, the adults who most often do stop to appreciate those little moments of beauty are those who realize that time is very limited—the very old and those who've had a brush with death. Neither group can pretend, as the rest of us too often do, that the song goes on forever. Knowing that it can end at anytime, they choose to listen to its melody while it's still playing.

And so should we.

Stop Weighting for a Miracle

A word of warning. Actually, it's a clarification. Media messages bombard us every waking hour—on the radio and television, in movies and magazines, even billboards—that equate better health with dieting. Well, the two are not synonymous.

Let's put it this way: Dieting is a short-term goal; good health is for a lifetime.

What happens typically is a woman realizes that an event such as her high school reunion, sister's wedding, or summer vacation is coming up, and she needs to lose twenty-two pounds before seeing her old friends, getting fitted for that gown, or wearing a bathing suit in public. So she turns to the latest fad diet, summons all her willpower, and reaches her target weight before the big occasion. Everyone tells her how great she looks. Then, almost immediately afterward, she begins her steady climb upward. Before she knows it she's gained all her weight back, and then some. Now she's got twenty-five pounds to lose and she's miserable.

Remember a few years ago when Oprah Winfrey announced, in front of the entire country, that she was going to fit into a pair of size ten jeans by a certain date? Armed with the willpower borne of potential embarrassment and possibly the loss of her credibility, she drank three protein shakes a day. Rarely did solid food pass her lips. To her way of thinking then, this massive exercise of willpower would sustain her into future encounters with food, enabling her to maintain the weight loss long after she hit her target. By then, she figured, she'd be able to eat sensible amounts of "real" food.

As almost everyone knows, at the end of the four-month diet, Oprah walked proudly across her stage wearing the size ten jeans while pulling a child's wagon filled with seventy-three pounds of simulated human fat—exactly the amount she'd lost on her diet.

Unfortunately, her results were as short-lived as her means were drastic. Soon she, too, gained back all the weight, until she came to terms with proper eating habits and regular exercise as the best solution to permanent weight loss.

There's nothing unique about Oprah's story. You may even have your own tale of the scale to tell. Maybe several of them. Because most people repeat the same mistake. Each time another special occasion presents itself, the process begins anew—and the failure cycle repeats. This time they decide to *really, really, really* exercise their willpower, or they change diets to the ultra-newest, or buy the latest and greatest piece of exercise equipment, vowing at every step to maintain the weight loss. By the end, the only thing they've lost is their common sense.

The greatest working definition of insanity I ever heard is, "Doing the same thing over and over while expecting the outcome to be different." That shoe fits chronic dieters, because approaching the problem with such temporary goals generates only temporary results. It always does. It always will. It's mainly for these reasons that the fitness industry has grown into a $9 billion business: It's fueled largely by people's desire for a quick fix—and quick fixes always fail, leaving the dieter to try another (quick fix) diet.

I'm not in the least suggesting that weight loss shouldn't be important to you if you're overweight. Nor am I telling you not to be concerned with prevailing standards of beauty. Though I'm not thrilled about it, I know that we're all affected to some degree by these images of "perfection" that we're bombarded with in the media.

The irony is that they're not selling better health; they're just selling an image. And we, unfortunately, buy into that. Most diet books, diet aids, and fitness equipment are bought by people who care only about improving their looks, not their health.

What do I mean by health? In this country, as in much of the world, health is unfortunately defined as the absence of illness. To me, that is the narrowest of definitions. Sure, not having the flu, not suffering with cancer or heart disease, being free of asthma's grip, are undeniably important goals. But health isn't necessarily just living without those diseases. It's bigger than that.

I consider health to be a state in which the body supports the kind of lifestyle that gives your life meaning and purpose. So if you

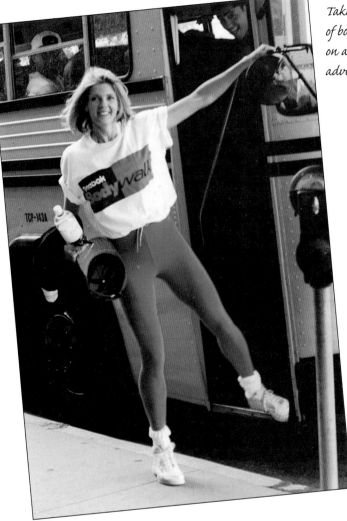

Taking a group of body walkers on a fitness adventure.

derive profound pleasure from going to the beach, or skiing, or taking long walks, or playing with your kids or grandchildren, then your body must be able to support these activities.

Until recently, too many so-called experts preached that lowered body fat automatically equated to good health. They wishfully believed that as all the weight came off, people would realize how much better they felt, which would quite naturally lead to a lifestyle change. But, given that thin itself was usually the target, there was no way to hit the good health bull's-eye.

The message had become, "You can look like this, and if you do, you'll have a better life." Nowhere, not even between the lines, was the message that you'll *feel* better. Not physically, anyway. You may feel better *about the way you look*, but good health and all of its gifts were left undiscussed.

And probably for good reason: Dieting does not make you feel good. Oh sure, you can get a burst of energy, even euphoria, for a few days here and there as the pounds burn. It's actually more of an adrenaline rush, realizing that the diet is "working." But if it really did make you feel good, then you wouldn't struggle so hard to stay on it. You wouldn't give it up so readily. You wouldn't have to call it a "diet."

Research has proven—and so have my common sense and experience—that dieting for the sole purpose of changing the way you look will always lead to disappointment: temporary weight loss followed by a usually bigger weight gain. On the other hand, the research also shows that when people lose weight gradually in order to *improve their health*, their pounds tend to stay off.

In other words, don't diet. Instead, approach weight loss in terms of a comprehensive plan of good health. While dieting may give you a ten-pound loss after a month, the odds are exceptionally high that you'll put back on all ten pounds and more within weeks after stopping the diet. Whereas if you go on a sensible regimen of moderating your calories and fat, building muscle, and conditioning yourself aerobically, the excess fat weight will get lost in good time. No, not as quickly as those crash diets. But by merging weight loss with an overall approach to good health—one in which you don't have to deprive yourself forever of all those foods you love, such as hot fudge sundaes and hamburgers—you're much more likely to arrive naturally at your target weight (unless it's unrealistically low) and stay there without undue effort.

Look, there are no quick fixes. I guarantee you that if you search carefully enough for the fine print under every extravagant claim made about weight loss, you'll find the words, "Works best when used in conjunction with a healthy diet and regular aerobic exercise."

There's no way to overemphasize the fact that dieting doesn't work. What does work is sensible eating and exercise.

Not long ago I received a beautiful but painful letter from a woman who took the time to describe in intimate detail her ongoing battle with weight loss and weight gain. She was a human yo-yo, with her emotions rising and falling as precipitously as her weight. The letter's last line said it all with such heartbreaking eloquence: "Kathy," she wrote, "send me a miracle."

Believe me, if I were capable of granting her that miracle, I would. But there is no miracle. No magic potion. No mysterious "thigh-away" cream that melts the inches while you sleep. No diet—whether it's all protein, all carbohydrate, or all celery—that will keep you at your goal once you get there.

People don't like to hear that. They prefer to wait around for the person, the product, the pill, the machine that will miraculously swoop down and rescue them from the body they inhabit.

Please, stop being one of those people. You are the genie in your own Aladdin's lamp, the one who can grant miracles and wishes. The power to do so has always been, and will always be, within you. You alone can change the life you have into the one you want.

THE POWER OF CHOICE PLAN

THE WHOLE IDEA OF "GETTING BETTER ALL THE TIME" MAY seem as unreal to you as an advertising slogan. You know what I mean: "You're not getting older, you're getting better," or "Life begins at forty (or fifty, etc.)." In other words, nothing more than words.

So let me assure you that getting better all the time is an absolutely attainable goal. All you have to do is choose it. And the way you do that is by following my Power of Choice Plan. It's a comprehensive, easy-to-understand, and easily accessible formula for taking control of your life—from relationships to fitness, exercise to eating—so that every day, in every way, you really do get better all the time.

PART ONE
THE POWER OF MIRACLES

THE MOMENT YOU CHOOSE TO BETTER YOUR LIFE IS THE MOMENT you choose good health instead of dieting. Such simple, concrete steps as eating properly and sensibly, and exercising regularly, begin paying off almost immediately with increased confidence and energy. You won't have to stand on the scale for validation. You'll see the results in every area of your life.

And as you continue your commitment to getting better, you'll have more strength and greater freedom. Instead of measuring your self-esteem by a number on the scale, you can choose to measure your success by the undeniable improvements in your relationships, your work, your family, and your productivity. But instead of waiting for that miracle to come along, you will have created it.

Creating miracles works for any area of your life, whether it's diet or exercise, work or social. You begin by taking three simple steps. First you set goals. Then you brainstorm solutions. And finally you take action steps. These three steps will help you to focus, to decide exactly what you want and need to make your life better. Once these three steps are taken, you can begin on the seven keys to success, which are the characteristics I've observed in others who have created their own miracles and made their dreams come true. Combining these three steps with the seven keys will ensure you success in achieving your goal of making your life better.

SET GOALS

People who spend time trying to understand the big picture of where they want to go in life are more likely to begin with a target, a goal, or a destination—the place they want to get to. Because if you don't know where you want to go, you can't complain when you get nowhere. Let's face it, it helps to have a plan to get where you're going.

I set goals all the time, work to reach them, then evaluate my strategy. I continue this process throughout the year. I even write my goals in a notebook so I can refer to them as a reminder. Goal setting is so important to me that it has evolved into an annual event. Let me explain.

The first of every new year, my husband, Steve, and I put the kids to bed, then gather in front of the fireplace with some close friends. Over two consecutive nights each of us lets down our defense mechanisms and admits out loud what he or she really wants out of life, no matter how odd or ridiculous it seems. Since we do this every year, we get a good glimpse of where we are today against the backdrop of where we wanted to be last year at the same time. It's like getting a report card on how we did in the last 365 days.

In other words, we begin each new year by setting goals.

The first night is always devoted to personal goals, the second night to professional goals. With a timer set for five minutes, we begin by writing down everything we'd like to accomplish personally in the year ahead. The magnitude of the goals or whether they're realistic is unimportant. What we're after is a completely uncensored list of our hearts' desires, compiled without fear of embarrassment or judgment. Fantasies or not, attainable or not, each item's presence represents a statement of possibilities.

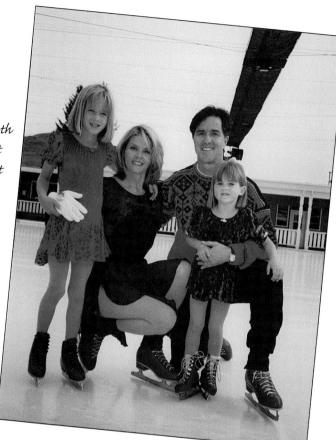

*Family Fitness.
Steve and I are both
from the Midwest
and we love to get
out on the ice.*

When the bell rings after five minutes, we then take some time to rate each item on a scale of importance, from one to five, five being most important. We then take all the "fives" and explain the importance of those goals in our lives. For example, if the goal is to lose weight, is it for self-esteem, better health, more energy? The object of this exercise is to be specific: Deciding how our lives would be improved if we realized that goal. The more specific you get, the more motivated you will become.

With the writing and the rating completed, we now begin sharing our goals with one another. This, for most of us, is the hardest part. It means getting over your fears of how others will react. However intimate you think you are with friends, letting them in on your deepest fantasies and desires takes some courage.

Interestingly, as difficult as it is to find the courage to admit your desires in front of the group, in many ways it's harder when you have to refrain from offering editorial commentary or explanation alongside each one. Such as: "I know I'll never be able to do this, but . . ." Or, "I know I've said this one before . . ." Or, "You may think I'm crazy, but . . ." The point is, you can't make your desires come true by constantly reminding yourself that they're only dreams.

Setting goals is the critical first step in creating your miracle. Stop now and grab a notebook or a few clean sheets of paper, and take a few minutes to write down your goals. Be specific and think about what's important to you. As we move through the process, you'll be able to refer back to your goals to identify solutions and create your action steps.

As an example, here's what my goals looked like for this year and how I ranked them. Notice how some goals were more important than others:

MY PERSONAL GOALS

Ranking	Goals
3	Learn how to use the Internet
5	Attend a couples workshop with my husband
2	Regular letter writing to friends
4	Learn Spanish
5	Run a 10-K in forty minutes
5	Start a foundation that helps girls get into sports
2	Cut back on chocolate
3	Take piano lessons
5	Make my life less chaotic at the end of the day
4	Coach my daughter's basketball team

To help you understand how the process works, let's focus on one of my fives: making my life less chaotic at the end of the day.

WHY IT'S IMPORTANT TO ME

Making my life less chaotic at the end of the day:
- The kids need to be picked up from after-school activities.
- They need my attention and help with their homework.
- There are chores to do in the kitchen, dinner to be prepared.
- The office usually has business issues that require my input, but they could wait till morning.

Now comes the time to take the next step: Figuring out how to achieve those goals. That means brainstorming solutions.

BRAINSTORM SOLUTIONS

I love to solve problems. It's not that I have any special talent for it as much as the proper attitude: I'm clear in my own mind that solving problems means asking the right questions. Whenever I can't find an answer for the problem at hand, I immediately go back to the question I'm asking and try to find a new question that will open up more options. I must do that ten times a day, for problems ranging from family relationships to business matters. In essence, I widen my perspective to include all the choices available, not just the one or two I'd originally focused on.

I guess you could say that, for me, brainstorming is a way of life. It's a process of spontaneously gathering ideas to find solutions to specific problems. It requires asking questions and allowing my mind to freely look at a situation without the constraints of reality and my own biases. In other words, anything is, and should be possible in the brainstorming process.

Remember my goal to make my evenings less chaotic? Here are some of the solutions I brainstormed:

1. Do food preparation earlier in the day.
2. Asking my husband to help with the kids.
3. Hiring a neighborhood girl to watch the girls.
4. Avoid business phone calls after hours.

In looking over my list, I realized that while my life in the evening hours was focused on home and family life, the constantly ringing telephones were actually my biggest source of aggravation, because they kept taking me away from what mattered most. It seemed the most obvious solution—and the simplest one—was to just turn off the phones between 5 and 7 P.M.

Here's another brainstorming example that came out of last New Year's session. One of the women in the group is a friend whose primary goal was to lose weight:

First, she listed all the reasons for doing so: She felt uncomfortable and unattractive, and didn't get as much accomplished as she needed to because of decreasing energy; in short, her life wasn't as vibrant as it used to be. Between taking care of the house and kids, husband and job, she had nothing left for herself. By the end of the day, every hour had been filled taking care of something or someone else. Though I empathized utterly with her feelings, I couldn't let her off the hook so easily. Saying you don't have the energy to take care of your health is akin to saying you're too far in debt to get a job.

"Exercise," I said.

"But I don't have time," she said.

So that's where we concentrated our brainstorming efforts, by dissecting her schedule. She and her husband got the kids ready in the morning. He dropped them off at school on his way to work. Meanwhile, she'd already left for her job as an accountant, but arranged time off to pick up the kids from school and get them to soccer practice two days a week. When practice ended, she rushed home and made dinner while the kids did homework. After dinner, she cleaned the kitchen. And after that, all she wanted to do was sit quietly, either reading a book or watching television.

We found two possible solutions. One was to have her husband get the kids ready for school by himself three mornings a week

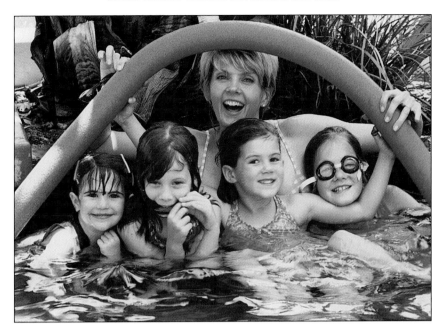

*Swimming and laughing with the girls and their friends
at Perrie's fifth birthday party.*

while she exercised for thirty minutes. The other was to power walk, maybe with the other moms, while their kids were at soccer practice; they could use the periphery of the field as a track, having the same conversations they would have had anyway while watching.

We went on and on like that for each person, brainstorming suggestions, some of which were usable, some of which weren't. But even the unusable ones were helpful, because they often gave the others a hint of information that could be turned into a brilliant suggestion. At a certain point, as always happens, we lost any sense of embarrassment or fear of ridicule for saying something stupid.

Go back now to the list of goals you created. Look at the number fives on the list and brainstorm solutions to your goals. Once you've brainstormed solutions, you're then ready to take action steps.

TAKE ACTION STEPS

Now it becomes time to take the steps that will make your dreams come true. Because setting goals doesn't much matter if you don't act on them.

I define action steps as doing whatever is required for you to accomplish your goal.

So if, for example, your goal is to lift weights every day, you have several choices. If you own weights, then you have to make time for them. If you don't own weights, then you either have to join a gym, buy some weights, or find someone who will let you use theirs.

It's incredibly helpful to write down your action steps. Very often, this is what separates actually doing them from just thinking about them. Make a list of the steps, such as 1) join a gym, 2) go every Monday, Wednesday, and Friday after work. Etc.

That's easy enough.

For more complicated or ambitious goals, I advise breaking the process down into smaller, more manageable steps. That way, the glow of passion is more likely not to fade under frustration.

Remember my goal of running a 10-K, and to complete it in forty minutes? That's a pretty lofty target if I haven't been training for a while. So instead of just white-knuckling it every day, I break down the process into small, doable steps—and write out each step on paper, something I can refer to. For one, I don't even think about running the full 6.2 miles. I begin by building my base—that is, for a month I only focus on running two miles three times a week. Then I increase the distance to three miles, then four, then five, and finally the six miles it will take. By the time I've gotten that far, I'm no longer overwhelmed by the task.

Ironically, I came upon this process by accident when I was running my first marathon in Hawaii, in 1975. At mile eighteen, I looked up and saw that monster, Diamond Head, facing me, taunting me. No way was I going to be able to get to its top and over the other side. I wanted to quit. Every fiber of my body and soul felt whipped. Luckily, though, a friend was running with me. "Just put one foot in front of the other," she said. "Forget about the finish line. Just one foot in front of the other. One step at a time."

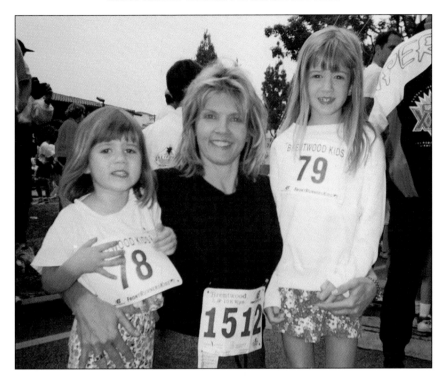

Brentwood 10-K is an annual tradition. This year Kate and Perrie ran the 1-K and then were there to cheer me across the 10-K finish line.

Well, I heeded her advice. Instead of having to run another eight miles, I thought of it as a series of absurdly short races—one-step races. All I had to do was take one more step, then another. And as a matter of fact, those final eight miles were the easiest of the whole marathon for me.

I never forgot that lesson. Anything can be broken down to small steps—action steps—that can be completed one little step at a time. In every aspect of life, no matter what your goal, remember that you can take small, doable steps. That's the way you build a bridge, write a book, lose weight, or change your life—step by step. If you find that you're not taking them, then either the steps weren't really doable, or you need to go back and check your motivation.

The more specific your action steps are, and the finer you can break them down into doable increments, the more successful you're going to be.

Seven Keys to Success

Okay. You've set goals for yourself, brainstormed ways to make them happen, and taken action steps toward actually turning them into reality. If you're like most people, you probably feel a sense of empowerment. And I hope you do, because seeing a plan to make dreams come true actually laid out before your eyes should be wonderfully hopeful and helpful.

Now I'm going to introduce you to the seven keys to success I've observed in people whose dreams do come true.

POWER OF CHOICE—
SEVEN KEYS TO SUCCESS

1. Make It a Priority
2. Be Consistent
3. Shift Your Mind-set
4. Find a Passion
5. Manage Stress
6. Keep a Diary
7. One Step at a Time

Key #1—MAKE IT A PRIORITY

Working with clients who wanted to lose weight or get in shape, I've noticed over the years that certain people can take the information and make it work for them, while others have huge stum-

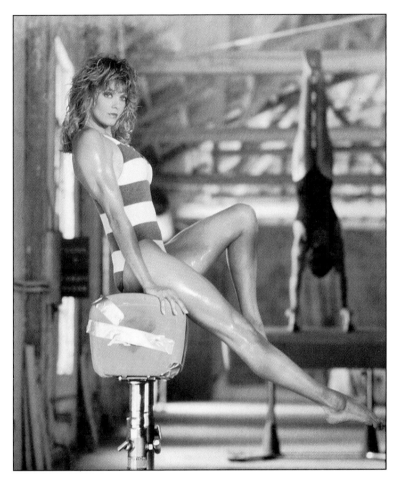

An ad for my Tickets leotard line in 1984.

bling blocks and excuses. I've heard them all: no time, lack of energy, sore back or knee, don't know what to do, confused, etc.

What's your excuse? Why don't you take better care of your health?
What's in the way of you discovering and maintaining self-esteem?

My experience has been that some people are able to make up
their minds to lose weight and exercise—they just do it. And some
people can't. I don't think it's a lack of willpower. It's just that some
people either fail to see the importance of getting healthy or they
feel that life has conspired against them.

The truth, though, is that people who've succeeded don't have more time or fewer problems. It's just that they've chosen to make good health a high enough priority; they've discovered ways of adjusting their schedules and lives in order to exercise and eat right.

There are plenty of days when I don't feel like putting in time on the treadmill or working out. But when I experience these thoughts, I immediately alter my perception. First, I think about how I'll feel after exercising. Next, I'll think about something a little different I could do that day to add variety to the workout, like putting on an old CD, say, Rod Stewart or The Beatles, which will take me on a trip down memory lane. Then I go into the ritual of putting on my shoes and workout clothes. Often, this is enough to stop the chatter in my mind. Instead of listening to "Oh, I'm tired, I don't feel like doing this," I shift to "I wonder if the weather will be nice tomorrow so we can go for a long hike." Or, "I wonder what I can do with the kids this weekend." Once you set your body in motion, you've won more than half the battle.

What also helps is to review all your reasons for wanting and needing to work out in the first place. When people come to me personally for weight-loss help, I insist that they write down their specific goals. For example: "I need to lose fifty pounds."

Why? I ask.

Usually a woman's first answer is, she wants to look better. But there are surface goals and inner-personal goals. The first is usually about wishes, the other about priorities. Surface goals tend to stand isolated from the bigger picture of life, so they're not as powerful in terms of motivation. The woman who answers, "I want to look better" won't be as motivated—and therefore stands a lesser chance of success.

On the other hand, the inner personal goals reflect real priorities. If you can get to the reasons *behind* wanting to look better, then there is a much greater chance of success. For instance, "Okay, I admit it. Every day when my kids come home I snap at them, because I'm so tired and short-tempered. My husband and I don't make love anymore because I don't feel good about myself. I look in the mirror every day and don't like the way my eyes look; they're saggy and make me look older than I am. I don't seem to have the confidence I used to have."

These words often carry the weight of a commandment. Your goal now isn't just thinner thighs or a tighter tummy. It's improving your entire life, and the way you feel about yourself.

If you really want something, and your reasons for it are strong enough, they will motivate you to make it a priority. They will be stronger than your inertia or your laziness.

Key #2—BE CONSISTENT

What's the secret to health and fitness success? That's the question I'm asked far more than any other.

The answer: Be consistent. Be consistent. Be consistent.

For more than twenty years, I've exercised every day. Now, does that mean full, hour-long workouts? No. Some days, in fact, I only have time for ten minutes; other days, only thirty; still others, a strenuous, two-hour hike. There are periods when I'm traveling for a week or so and only able to get in a few minutes of exercise between meetings. But whether it's ten minutes, thirty, or a long sixty, I make sure I work up as much of a sweat as possible. Not only because I'm trying to burn off last night's dinner or because I think it'll improve my cardiovascular capacity, but because I don't want to fall out of practice. That's what I mean by consistency—if you fall out of the habit, get right back on track.

Often when I talk to people who aren't exercising on a consistent basis, I get the feeling that they have the best intentions, but allow one excuse after the next to interfere with their workouts. Then, they lose momentum. "I was exercising and then all of a sudden I just stopped," is a common lament. "I don't know what happened; I just sort of quit. I haven't really done it for six months, but I plan on starting again right after my birthday."

But exercise and self-care is not an on-and-off proposition. It's a daily one. If you don't have time to do your regular workout in its entirety you don't abandon the whole thing. That's not the way to approach exercise.

Try thinking of it this way. You have a goal—an ideal, if you will. The ideal is to work out five times a week for at least thirty minutes. But if you can't get in all thirty, then you take what you can. That's the way life works. Just because you fall short of an ideal doesn't mean that you abandon its pursuit. Telling a single lie wouldn't compel you to give up honesty as an ideal any more than accidentally running a red light causes you to break every other rule of the road.

The hardest aspect of exercise is starting again after not doing it for a while. That's why I try not to lose my momentum—so I don't have to start all over again.

Just accept that you'll devote at least ten minutes a day to exercising, the same as you accept that you're going to have to eat, bathe, and dress. Now, those ten minutes may not necessarily be at the gym or on the track. They may be that walk you take by parking a little farther away from the office. Or the stairs you climb instead of pushing the elevator buttons.

Once you choose to make exercise a daily part of your life, you start to see opportunities for it where before you saw only barriers. That viewpoint begins to create lifestyle changes, and produces a healthier attitude toward life in general.

Consistency also applies to eating—which is another question I'm often asked: How do you have the willpower to be good all the time?

Answer: I don't think in terms of good or bad. As we'll discuss in depth in Part Two of my plan, I eat in a way that serves me, my health, and my body. And that includes eating all kinds of foods, some of which many people may consider "bad."

If I had to explain it in terms of "good" and "bad," I'd say that you only have to be "good" 80 percent of the time. That allows you, pretty much, to do whatever you want with the other twenty and still not upset the equation. You can splurge on a Nestlé's Crunch bar. Indulge your craving for Ben & Jerry's. Give in to the tempting smell of apple pie. Just be consistently on track the other 80 percent of the time.

By the same token, the 80-20 rule frees you from the trap of thinking that just because you ate four potato chips, you might as well eat the whole bag.

For instance, when I was pregnant with my first daughter, Katie,

I developed the strongest craving for bacon, lettuce, and tomato sandwiches. While this might not seem strange to you, I'd not eaten a piece of bacon for fifteen years. And yet, I could sit down and eat not one but two BLTs at a single meal. Concerned, I checked with my doctor, who assured me that the craving was normal, and perhaps I needed a little more salt in my diet.

After Katie was born, I fortunately lost the craving for bacon. Unfortunately, I've never lost my craving for chocolate. This is an ongoing issue for me. In fact, I'm learning to control my relationship with chocolate. I allow myself to eat it once a week—no guilt, no shame, no worry. The other days, I nibble on fresh fruit, or homemade rice pudding, or suck on a piece of hard candy to satisfy my sweet tooth. I've also learned not to keep large quantities of chocolate around the house. If there were, I'd be tempted to nibble on it every day. I know myself. Giving myself permission to indulge has taken chocolate out of the "bad" food category—and it's no longer an obsession.

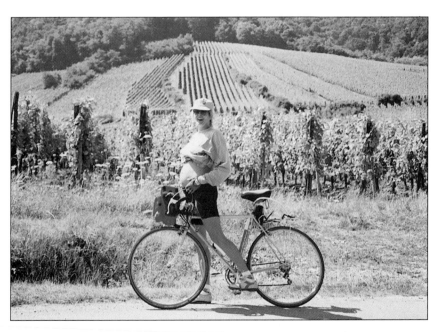

Cycling through the vineyards of France was quite an adventure.
I was pregnant with Katie, who would always
let me know when it was time to rest.

I feel a sense of calm about my eating habits. I never feel deprived, and I don't like to listen to someone talk about calories or fat grams when I'm eating. My attitude is, when you're eating, enjoy. And when you're satisfied, stop.

That's what I tell people when they ask for my health and fitness secrets. I tell them, the secret is consistency. The three-month give-it-all mentality is only good for players in the Super Bowl. But when it comes to developing a healthy lifestyle, it's a day in, day out, week in, week out, year in, year out game plan that leads to success.

Key #3—SHIFT YOUR MIND-SET

I remember once picking up an old photo album from the coffee table and thumbing through the pictures of my childhood. This time, the captioned dates and locations caught my attention. In 1951 I was in Arizona; 1952, Oklahoma; 1953, San Diego; 1956, Brazil; 1959, Alabama; 1963, Hawaii; 1966, Illinois. Change had been a way of life back then. Every time I made friends, got attached to a house or my bedroom in it, or bonded with a teacher, my dad would announce that it was time to pack up and move. Such was the life of an air force family. I accepted it as the way things were. I would walk into each new school wondering which of those faces belonged to my new best friend. Though I was young and just doing what came naturally, I think now that I'd somehow made a conscious decision to be optimistic and to make the best of the situation.

Being flexible, being open, shifting your mind-set, is a powerful choice. And because it doesn't always look like a choice, people often miss it.

Successful people adopt the proper attitude to react to ever-changing circumstances. They know that how and what they picture in their mind will create the mood they're in and the kind of behaviors that follow. Successful people have shown that the quality of life is determined not by what happens to them, but rather by what they do about what happens.

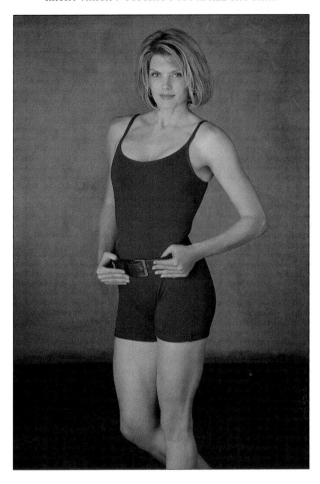

For instance, being able to work out effectively at the end of the day will depend on what sort of mood you're in and how you picture that workout in your mind. If for hours ahead of time you've been dreading going to the gym because, say, you don't like the clothes you brought to work out in, or you can't bear to see that gorgeous blonde who always wears a skimpy leotard so that all the men will stare at her, you'll produce a certain state of mind that, frankly, isn't exactly conducive to going to work out. On the other hand, if you're looking forward to meeting your girlfriend there and finding out all about her new job, or you can't wait to take your favorite instructor's aerobics class, you'll produce a totally different state of mind—and, thus, behaviors. Obviously, you behave differently when angry or anxious than you do when you're excited. So you're less likely to have a good workout when negative feelings intrude.

It's an endless cycle. Because when you do have a great workout, and begin to feel physically vibrant, you perceive the world differently—with more love and enthusiasm. And that, of course, creates a mind-set to take care of yourself.

The key to getting to the gym, or to wherever you work out, consistently is to represent things to yourself in such a way that you're going to want to take positive action. In short, you have to be in charge of filtering your thoughts throughout the day.

Sometimes, though, that's difficult. For me, it happens when I'm tired. I experience such a dramatic change in my thought patterns compared to when I've had a good night's sleep that things begin looking sour to me. Instead of looking forward to new challenges, I start dreading every commitment on my calendar. Each question I'm asked can no longer be answered simply, because I read more sinister, ulterior meanings into the words.

So, knowing this about myself, I've learned that if I don't get enough sleep, I can't keep my mind shifted into the positive direction that serves me best. If I stay up too late, I'm less likely to get up at 6 A.M., full of life and ready to work out.

My attitude is that I'm in charge of what I think and how I interpret events, so I pay attention to the chatter in mind, and when it starts bad-mouthing the world, I respond accordingly. I shift my mind-set to keep me on track, especially where my health and fitness are concerned.

Key #4—FIND A PASSION

Why is it that when we fall in love or are excited about an opportunity, we seem to enjoy boundless energy and can go for days with very little sleep?

The reason is passion.

A few years ago when I was watching a PBS series hosted by Bill

Moyers, it caught my attention when the great mythologist Joseph Campbell urged us to follow our "bliss." Because that's what I've done in my life. I follow my bliss, which I interpret to mean passion, and I encourage you to find and follow your own.

I once read a fascinating report on longevity that discussed a study of 100 people who were then in their nineties or older. The study's author said that he could find only two traits common to all 100 people. The first, that they'd eaten a consistent diet their entire lives, meaning that they'd had no extreme weight losses or gains. But it was the second trait that most captured my attention: All the old people were extremely interested in something outside themselves, whether it was religion, a hobby, or volunteering, etc. In other words, they'd found a passion.

In the early 1980s I began putting together everything I'd ever learned about exercise, fitness, and health into teaching an aerobics class in the San Fernando Valley. Though my pay was only about ten dollars per class, I considered myself incredibly rich and successful. Why? Because every day some woman, age thirty to fifty, would come up to me and admit, with tears in her eyes, that since reaching adulthood she hadn't moved her body the way she was doing in my class; she thought she'd forgotten how. But now, after sticking with it for several months, she'd begun to feel her entire life change. "I've decided I'm going to go out and get a job," was a common statement of joy. Others bragged that sex with their husbands had picked up again after a long layoff.

I could see that I was impacting these women, that their self-confidence had been raised and their well-being improved. The first step had been moving their bodies, the next—well, who knows.

Later, I became the cohost of a USA Cable show called *Alive & Well*, on which I led a daily mini-class of exercise. Suddenly, I began receiving thousands of letters that echoed the sentiments of these women who'd come up to me in class. Heartfelt letters, describing the enormously positive changes they were experiencing.

To tell you the truth, the reason I continue to do what I do in my professional life (including writing this book) is that I'm committed to helping people. Nothing gives me more pleasure than to hear that, for whatever reason, I've inspired someone to consider today the first day of the rest of her life. As I noted before, I save each and every letter. And the in-person exchanges remain indelibly imprinted in my memory.

I remember an appearance at a store in Minneapolis's Mall of America. A man and his nineteen-year-old daughter waited in line for an hour to tell me their story. It seems that, two years before, the daughter had decided to drop out of high school because of depression, feeling that her life was worthless. Distraught over his daughter's decision, about which he could do nothing legally since she was past sixteen, the father tried every form of persuasion, even bribery. Nothing worked. Then one day he happened to see a

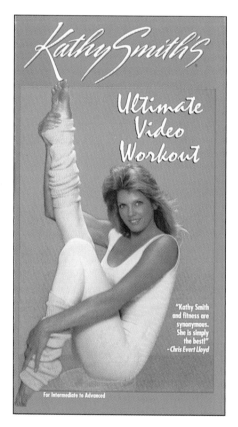

The cover of my first video. I was thirty-two years old.

poster of mine that read, BELIEVE IN YOURSELF. He bought it along with one of my exercise videos and brought them home to her. Resistant at first, she tried the video, then hung the poster. Within weeks, she'd exercised out the depression and taken the slogan to heart. She stayed in school, graduated, and was, when I met her, enjoying her freshman year of college. Both father and daughter had tears in their eyes, and so did I.

Handing me both the poster and the video, the daughter said, "You made me believe I could do it, that I could do something with my life."

As we hugged and exchanged tissues, I understood the emotional connection between us: We both shared a passion for exercise, and she, like me, now understood that it had expanded her options by allowing her to notice more opportunities, and to take better advantage of them, which is exactly what it has done for me.

If she'd asked me to explain to her the cause and effect of exercise and its results, I would have said that, as scientific research has demonstrated, exercise has a generally healthy effect on the human mind and spirit, as well as the body.

Now, does exercise automatically lead to major life changes for everyone? No, probably not.

Personally, I've found that my thinking is often at its most creative when I'm working out—whether running, walking, lifting weights, treadmilling, riding the Exercycle, etc. It's a conscious choice, to use the time productively. I'm fully aware that a lot of people abandon their exercise programs because they get bored. They lose their passion.

"Don't you?" they ask.

Lose my passion? Never. First of all, I don't let myself get to that point; I cross-train, moving from one activity to another nearly every day. Second, I don't get bored because there's so much to think about when I'm exercising. Sure, the activity itself can be repetitive, but that very repetition frees the mind to go elsewhere.

Exercise initiates physiological reactions that also lead to subtle changes in thought processes. In the calm of an exercise-induced alpha state, I trust my mind to be more agile, so I tend to follow where it wants to lead. During exercise, my mental state reflects the best of me from the deepest recesses of my soul.

Even when I don't need to solve a particular problem, I often use the time to take stock of my life: Am I being a good mother? A good wife? A good employer? A good role model? Am I treating those around me well? How can I be better?

Other times, I spend my workout enjoying some detailed day-dreaming such as getting lost in nature—enjoying the sights, smells, and sounds. And finally, I also brainstorm solutions to problems at home or work during my workout. Often this brainstorming will lead to some creative solutions.

Now all these years later, I still revel in my passion for exercise. Being connected passionately to one thing leads to other areas of passion, including one for life in general. You then naturally want to experience more, be more involved in life. You develop a healthier lifestyle, and that means not having to focus so single-mindedly on food, your weight, your body image, your finances, or whatever.

I encourage you to nurture a passion for fitness, and let that passion connect you to other dreams and other passions. From art to cooking to gardening to travel, let exercise be your guide.

Whatever your dreams, follow their trail. Go where they lead. Listen to your heart. Chase your passions.

Key #5—MANAGE STRESS

Life is inherently stressful. Both at work and at home, stressful situations are everywhere. Always have been, always will be. What we do with that stress, though, is up to us. What I've found is that learning to cope with stress effectively is a major component of success.

We use the word stress so often, we don't even stop to think about its meaning. So what is stress?

Scientists tell us that stress is simply our body's response to change. The key word is "response," because stress itself is neither positive nor negative. It's the *quality* of our response to stress that makes it positive or negative.

Stress causes a response in our bodies and the production of certain chemicals that prepare us for action. What kind of response? Well, to name a few, our heart rate jumps, our blood pressure increases, our eyes dilate, we perspire, our muscles tense.

What's happening is that our sympathetic nervous system, *without our control*, is reacting to perceived danger.

This is the same basic system that protected cavemen from woolly mammoths. And today the system still works wonderfully when we need to, let's say, jump out of the path of an oncoming truck.

But it's not so great when you start seeing your spouse as a woolly mammoth. Your stress reaction is out of control.

Stress doesn't just occur around major life crises—such as a death in the family, or a divorce. In this day and age, the situations that cause stress are more likely to be everyday occurrences. Juggling two jobs, paying bills and dealing with taxes, a traffic jam, worries about crime, deadlines at work, family responsibilities— these are all factors that cause our bodies to start reacting, making us human time bombs, ready to explode.

Yes, life will always give us stress. So you must understand that it's how we manage it that counts. Now I say "manage" and not "eliminate." That's because a little stress—like a little chocolate— can be a good thing. It energizes you to get your work done. In fact a study by Harvard scientists clearly demonstrated that at certain levels, stress improved job performance. But with too much stress, performance suffered.

So the trick is to manage stress, instead of stress managing you, because *anything* you do to reduce stress levels will improve your health.

TIPS FOR MANAGING STRESS

1. **Shoot for Sixes.** I'm a firm believer that we need to lower our expectations. We can't always score tens in life nor expect those around us to be perfect either. Lower the bar.

2. **Walk with a Friend.** There's compelling new research that confiding in a trusted friend about problems is one of the best ways to lower stress. So what better way to share time and thoughts, than on a walk with a friend?

3. **Eat Smart.** The other area doctors immediately turn to when dealing with stress is your diet. And no wonder. Excess caffeine, alcohol, and sugar all send the wrong message to your body. Eat smart to reduce stress.

4. **Deep Breathing.** There is no better way to get out of a stress attack than to practice deep breathing techniques. And it follows that regular meditative breathing is also an excellent way to avoid getting stressed out.

I practice all these tips myself on a regular basis. I love to share walks and workouts with friends and family—and find my husband and I often have our most meaningful conversations while taking our evening walks. Of course, I've learned over the years about the benefits of a healthy diet and know my eating habits have helped lower my stress. And finally, there is not a day in my life that I don't take time for myself and practice my breathing technique. Sometimes it's as little as two minutes. Other days I might use this breathing technique for up to twenty minutes. Deep, meditative breathing is an essential part of my life.

Coincidentally, deep breathing is also an essential part of exercise. When you work out strenuously, you breathe deeply. Any aerobic workout increases your oxygen demands, which are satisfied by deep breaths. But I want you to realize that you can use breathing throughout the day, to help relieve stress and provide a sense of calm. It's an incredibly effective way to get yourself centered and relaxed. No matter what else is going on—work demands, kids screaming, deadlines—when my stress level is high I'll stop what I'm doing for a minute, close my eyes, and follow the simple breathing technique I've devised.

How does it work? Like this. I inhale through my nose, trying to consciously direct air toward my expanding diaphragm. I then exhale slowly but completely out of my nose. Taking four or five deep breaths like that in succession can literally chase the craziness out of my body. With each successive breath, I became calmer.

And just the way exercise pays off dividends even after your workout by tinkering with your metabolism, so, too, over time, this deep breathing technique works its magic on your nervous system. Before long you'll notice a marked increase in your ability to calm down, quickly and efficiently.

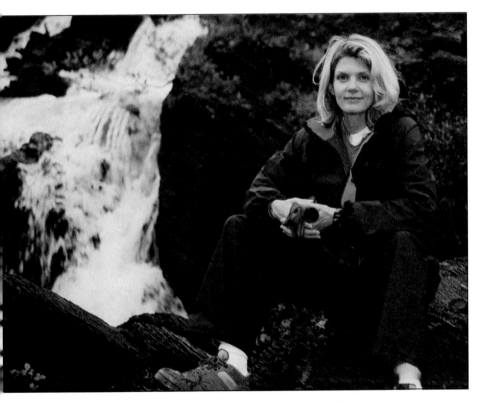

Glacier Park, Montana. I love rejuvenating myself by exploring the natural wonders all around us.

Deep breathing is free, it's easy, it doesn't require any special preparation, and it pays off with immediate rewards. How will you know for yourself? Only by trying the breathing technique.

I guarantee you a moment (and then a life) of calm.

KATHY'S STRESS-FREE BREATHING TECHNIQUE

1. *Relax your body.* Find a comfortable place to sit. Close your eyes. Relax your neck and shoulders (the places you hold stress) as best you can.

2. *Inhale through your nose.* On the inhale, fill your lungs so your diaphragm expands completely. Think of your belly as a balloon you're trying to inflate. The air should feel as if it's filling your entire body.

3. *Exhale through your nose.* It should feel like you're slowly releasing the air from a balloon.

4. *Keep it slow.* Match the speed of the inhale with the speed of the exhale. Don't breathe in fast and out slow and vice versa. Easy and steady both in and out.

5. *Expand the breath.* When you get comfortable with breathing this way, try and lengthen both parts of your breath. Keep your eyes closed, and relax.

There's no reason to be stretched to the breaking point in your day-to-day life. You can regain control of every situation and reduce your stress level by practicing this deep breathing technique.

Key #6—KEEP A DIARY

I love diaries. Always have. They're incredibly useful tools for change.

People generally think of diaries as a way of recording secret thoughts and feelings for posterity; that's why diaries often come with a little lock and key. But I've used them extensively for the good they can do today, and I'm not confining that to mean just the emotional and psychic release of expressing yourself without inhibition—though that's certainly worth something, too.

Let's say you've been trying to lose weight, and you just can't seem to figure out why the pounds aren't dropping off. You believe that you're eating well and exercising frequently enough—all the things you know you're supposed to do. So it's a mystery why you've remained at the same weight, or have even gotten heavier. Well, the solution to that mystery may lie in a diary.

Keeping a diary is an exercise in honesty. Your diary will give you tremendous insight into your own habits. We all say, "I should eat less fat." But do you have any idea of how much fat you're eating now? We all say, "I should work out more." But do you have any idea how many calories you've burned this week? Your diary will enable you to pinpoint exactly where you need to concentrate your efforts. Maybe you're consistent with your toning workouts, but you're letting your cardiovascular exercise slide. Maybe your fat intake is just fine, but you're eating too many calories. In order to make appropriate changes in your habits, you first need to know what your habits are. This means that you would, on a daily basis, keep a log of everything you eat and every exercise you perform, including its duration. After a week or two, a quick glance at the diary will give you some perspective on your eating and exercise habits.

I'll be introducing you to a food plan in Part Two, and keeping a diary will no doubt help with your success.

Diaries come in many shapes and forms. You can purchase a diary at most bookstores, or simply use a spiral-bound notebook for all your entries. Here's a sample page from my diary:

SAMPLE FROM KATHY'S DIARY— APRIL 29

TIME	FOOD	EXERCISE/ACT.	REMARKS
7:00 A.M.	orange, sliced oatmeal nonfat milk chopped almonds raisins		Made time for meditation before breakfast
8:30-9:30 A.M.		walk/run, stretch	
10:00 A.M.	banana protein shake		
noon	sliced turkey sandwich carrot sticks corn chips		Really rushed; no time; schedule too tight
4:00 P.M.	sweet potato topped with plain yogurt		
5:00 P.M.		shoot baskets with kids	
6:00 P.M.	rice and bean burrito avocado, chopped tomatoes, corn, salsa		Enjoyed dinner with family; discussed summer vacation
8:00 P.M.	nonfat yogurt with fresh raspberries cup of tea		

You might be surprised by what you learn. I sure was. I'm always preaching to my friends about the importance of calcium. My diary helped me discover *I* was the one short on calcium! It seemed like I was eating a cup of yogurt every day, but in fact I was only having it three times a week. Now yogurt is my regular afternoon snack.

I no longer keep a diary every day of my life, but it's a tool I often turn to when my weight starts creeping up. It's quite a wake-up call. Sometimes, I get into a phase where I grab a handful of walnuts every time I walk by the fridge. When I'm forced to record this in my diary, I say, "My gosh! That's thirty-three grams of fat—and I wasn't even hungry." Your diary will make you aware of "sub-snacks," the foods you don't even realize you're eating.

We all have ways of fooling ourselves; we convince ourselves that if we don't look at the package, those cookies *can't* be loaded with fat! Whether you're eating too much fat, skimping on fiber, or neglecting to exercise, your diary will hold you accountable.

Of course, diaries aren't just for dieting and exercise. They can be used to effect change in any other area of your life, because in order to change you must first know where you actually stand; only then can you choose to move somewhere else.

By keeping you honest, and forcing you to confront truths, diaries help you locate causes and their effects. You'd be surprised at how few people are really aware of what pushes their emotional buttons, and at how powerful it can be to develop that awareness.

Example: During my late twenties and early thirties, I'd often get the same unpleasant sensation, a tightness in the shoulders and neck, like the weight of the world was on me. With the help of psychologist Dr. Leslie Pam, I was able to eventually verbalize—and of course record in my diary—that I'd felt I had too many responsibilities and no one to turn to at the time.

Leslie taught me that when "something comes up" that wants to push me off kilter—in my case, the crushing responsibility in my professional or personal life, instead of turning to food and overeating—to stop for a moment, close my eyes, and ask myself what I'm feeling. Then I would write down my thoughts in my diary. It's necessary to be specific about them. *When have I felt this way before? Are there physical symptoms? Where are they located?* By doing this, I started to distinguish real hunger from anxiety. And even if I didn't find the source of anxiety right away, I just kept trying until I did.

Having to make daily diary entries about what you eat, how much you exercise, and what you're feeling forces you to face each day honestly. The entries don't have to be long and wordy—and they don't have to be recorded in an elaborate, leather-bound volume. A few thoughts on these three key areas, entered in a notebook (with the date above each entry), will suffice.

Those few important lines a day soon become a valuable document that can tell you much more about your life—that is, exactly where you are now—than virtually anything else. It's a bit like missing the forest for the trees: In the buzz of daily life, we're often unaware of how our behavior falls into patterns—how we repeat the same mistakes.

And as you progress, nothing will inspire you more than seeing your own triumphs in writing. It's documented proof of all your hard work!

Key #7—ONE STEP AT A TIME

I can still hear you thinking that things can't change for the better; that, without the magic wand, you're stuck in the body you have. So how can I convince you that you're entirely capable of choosing to make these positive changes?

What I'm going to do is show you how health and fitness totally impact key areas of your life. Let's look at them:

- general disposition
- family
- intimate relationships
- friendships
- work
- energy level
- appearance

Our general disposition is our calling card. It announces to the world who we are and tells the universe what we can expect to get. If we act grouchy and cranky, we can't expect to be treated any differently. But if we have a sunny disposition, which is what a fit, healthy person projects, we're more likely to attract goodness to ourselves.

The way we interact with our family is another gauge of our personality. While being tired often makes us indifferent, even destructive, feeling healthy and energized can help support the kind of loving, nurturing, family environment you dream of.

It's the same with our intimate relationships. Ask yourself whether your love life is satisfactory, pleasurable, worthwhile. Does it sustain you, give you the nourishment to attack the world outside? Is it a haven, a shelter? Is your sex life something to brag about? If, on the other hand, you're not currently in a love relationship, ask yourself why not. Would you like to be? What are you doing, then, to find the person you want to be with?

Our friendships are, in many ways, mirrors of who we are. The people we choose to surround ourselves with for fun and recreation, for companionship and company, reflect our values and interests. Do we make the time, have the energy, and express the enthusiasm to develop the kinds of friends we want? Or do we settle for less than the best because we lack energy, motivation, and self-esteem?

Ah, work. Do you enjoy it? Or do you feel like a beast of burden, spending half your time at work fantasizing being somewhere else? Do you contribute all you can? Are you moving forward at a pace you'd like? Is your work something you would do for free, or would you feel underpaid no matter how much you earned doing it?

Energy level may be the best overall indicator of our mental and physical health. When we wake up in the morning with a recharged battery, anxious to get at the day, it indicates that most if not all of the above categories fall on the plus side of life's ledger. But when we drag through the hours, relying on coffee or other stimulants to keep us moving, it says that we're not functioning at the highest level of involvement; we're less than we can be. And we're probably watching others lead the kind of life we'd like to lead.

Finally, appearance. Much like our general disposition, the way we look answers a lot of questions about our health and fitness. Is your body fit and healthy, or does it show signs of neglect?

I raise these issues to convince you that fitness affects every aspect of your life. And you have the power to improve your life by changing your relationship to health and fitness—one step at a time. Let your feet lead the way. It doesn't matter what diets or programs you've failed at in the past. We'll leave them there, where they belong. Forget about any therapies or self-help groups you may have tried and abandoned for lack of success. Put aside your skepticism. All the evidence you need is right in front of you: Changing nearly every aspect of your life—becoming who you'd like to be— is as easy as making a choice. That's all.

You can do it! You have the power!

Just remember, everything we want to accomplish takes time, especially when the goal is such a profound one. After all, if it didn't take time and patience, if it could be done at the snap of a finger, then it wouldn't be as worth it. Achieving good health and an optimum weight is not a concrete goal that can be reached as easily as multiplying two times two, because factors change constantly in our lives; we have to understand that the process is ongoing; it never ends. We're always fine-tuning and adjusting for circumstances.

Of course, this shift in thinking takes time and patience. Having patience with ourselves makes the whole process so much more fun. We aren't fixated on having something happen immediately. We let it unfold naturally, one step at a time, until eventually we have developed a new habit. Of this, I'm absolutely certain. As proof, I have the letters in my files, thousands of them, from women and men just like you who took the plunge and found that they got used to the water very quickly; every aspect of their lives improved.

So don't lose faith, even when you feel you have none to lose. Just keep putting one foot in front of the other, one step at a time. Follow the program and good things will happen.

PART TWO
THE POWER OF FOOD

ENJOYING YOUR FOOD

Wouldn't it be great to know you could eat just about anything and still accomplish all of your nutrition goals? And wouldn't it be even greater still to eat those foods and feel wonderful?

Well, it's entirely possible—and it's the goal of my food plan.

I've come to realize two important facts about food. First, foods that satisfy me and those that nourish me differ from day to day and meal to meal. Second, I've discovered that trying to follow a strict, you-can-eat-this-you-can't-eat-that diet is self-defeating; and flexibility is as important in eating and food choices as it is in exercise.

Of course, it's also important that food provide me with the fuel I need to feel good, and the nutrients my body needs to stay healthy. But there's one more thing:

I also want to enjoy my food.

In fact, I *need* to enjoy my food. The anticipation of it. Seeing the foods prepared. Admiring them on the plate. Those first few tastes. Chewing. Swallowing.

Food has always been—and will always be—a source of profound pleasure. I love the crunch of an apple, the texture and smell of warm bread, the savoriness of roasted chicken. I delight in the cool sweetness of ice cream and the absolute ecstasy of chocolate cake.

And I want to enjoy my food in a variety of settings. I cherish the meals my family and I share in our kitchen as much as I do great meals prepared in restaurants. In other words, I love food, and I love to eat.

What I've learned about food reflects what I've learned about life in general. My food has to be both functional and flexible. It has to meet my nutritional needs, while allowing my choices to vary day to day, based on the circumstances of that day. They're definitely not based on rigid guidelines. I don't choose my food because it's "nonfat" or allegedly "not fattening" and I don't choose food just because it's "good for me."

I choose my foods because I've worked to understand how food serves me—physically, mentally, and emotionally. And after reading this book, you'll have the tools to choose your foods so that they serve you as well. I want you to gain a greater understanding of your body and how your food choices affect you.

You can become a "functional" eater by learning to assess your needs at any given moment and choosing foods that meet those needs. This is something most of us are not used to doing. Either we get lazy and don't want to think about what we eat, or we get disciplined and go on a diet and have other people tell us what to eat.

I'd like to introduce you to a different approach. This approach is about you and for you. It focuses on what you need to eat and what you want to eat. It's about choices and the flexibility we all need in order to be consistent.

Surprisingly, consistency is not about rigidity. Which means that there's no such thing as "cheating." If you do "slip," all you do is get back on track as soon as possible—and eventually you find yourself slipping less and less.

When you blend consistency with my plan's built-in choices and flexibility, you get a truly functional approach to food and eating. You'll learn how to incorporate food into your life in a way that makes sense for your body and the way you live.

In the following section you'll read about the nutrients: carbo-hydrate, protein, and fats, as well as vitamins, minerals, and water. This information will help you to make your own intelligent, healthy decisions. I want you to be in control and know what these nutrients do in your body, for your body, and in which foods to find them.

Perrie and I in our best balancing act.

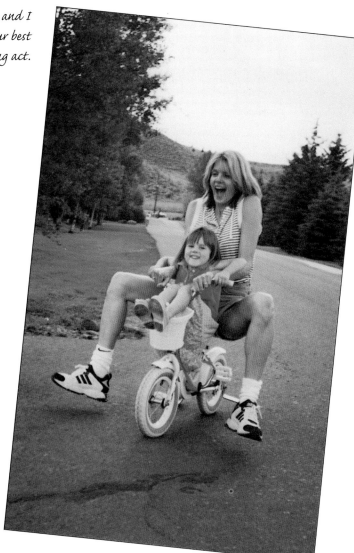

The Nutrients

A body that receives adequate nutrients gets the essentials for life, and is therefore considered to be properly nourished.

Nutritionists identify six primary groups of essential nutrients: carbohydrates, proteins, fats, vitamins, minerals, and water.

The six nutrient categories can be split into two separate groups for purposes of discussion. Carbohydrates, protein, and fat are called the energy nutrients. These are the only nutrients the body can metabolize for energy, which is typically measured in calories.

The second group—vitamins, minerals, and water—are essential components of our organs, skeletal structures, and other tissues, as well as hormones and enzymes that regulate specific body functions. Despite what you may believe, vitamins and minerals cannot give you extra energy, but do get involved in the process of metabolizing energy. Carbohydrates, protein, and fat are our only good sources of energy.

Think of the three energy nutrients as fuel and of vitamins and minerals as fuel enhancers; meanwhile, water is the system's lubricant. While you need fuel to function, vitamins, minerals, and water help you to function better.

The incredible number of foods we eat have one thing in common. They all contain some mix of carbohydrate, proteins, and fat. This mix is called food composition.

Food Composition

Everyone knows the old joke about feeling hungry again a few minutes after eating Chinese food. Well, as it turns out, there's a good reason for that phenomenon. The mix of carbohydrates, proteins, and fats you eat in a meal has a powerful impact on how long you feel satisfied after eating. Understanding food composition will help you to establish eating patterns that serve your choice to live better.

Carbohydrates and fats are the primary nutrients from which the body derives energy. Protein's more important function is the building and repairing of body tissues; it is converted to energy only when the other sources are unavailable. That's why people on restrictive diets lose muscle mass. The body has no choice but to target protein for fuel when there is not enough carbohydrate in the diet. When that happens, the protein is then unavailable for its primary use, and the body not only loses muscle mass but doesn't have protein available to rebuild the lost muscle tissue.

While the body can most readily convert carbohydrates into energy, all carbohydrates are not created equal. They are divided into two categories: simple and complex. The simplest carbohydrates found in refined sugars—juices, sodas, and jelly beans, for example—get into your bloodstream the quickest and are metabolized faster than complex carbohydrates. Complex carbohydrates are found in starches, whole grains, legumes, fruits, and vegetables. These carbohydrates contain fiber and are often a mix of both simple and complex carbohydrates.

CARBOHYDRATE FOOD SOURCES

Carbohydrates are quickly digested and metabolized. Simple carbohydrates such as sugar may keep you satisfied for as little as thirty minutes. Complex carbohydrates with starch and/or fiber may last up to two hours (depending on the number of calories consumed).

Simple Carbohydrates	Complex Carbohydrates
table sugar	fruit
honey	vegetables
syrups (including corn syrup)	breads, cereals

Simple Carbohydrates	Complex Carbohydrates
sodas and fruit drinks	bagels, muffins
refined fruit juices	grains such as rice, barley
most no-fat cookies, desserts	pasta, noodles
hard candy, jelly beans	potatoes, yams
sorbet, Popsicles	beans, legumes

When you eat a high-fiber diet you typically feel satisfied longer than when you eat the same number of calories from sugar. But even a meal of stir-fry vegetables and steamed rice can leave you feeling hungry within hours.

Adding a significant protein source to a meal can help us stay satisfied longer for two reasons: Protein takes longer to digest, and your body's response to protein helps to keep blood glucose levels elevated longer—so you'll feel satisfied longer.

PROTEIN FOOD SOURCES

A mix of protein and carbohydrate in a meal can keep you satisfied about three to four hours. You may find a difference between animal and vegetable sources of protein (depending on the number of calories consumed).

Animal Protein Sources	Vegetable Protein Sources
beef, lamb, other red meats	beans such as pinto and navy
chicken, turkey, other game	legumes such as lentils
fish and seafood	nuts and seeds
pork and pork products	nut butters (peanut butter)
milk, yogurt, cheese	soy beans and tofu
eggs	hydrolyzed vegetable protein

But if you want that feeling to last even longer, include some fat in the meal. That's right. Eat fat! Fat triggers the release of hormones that slow down the digestive process. Your blood glucose will remain elevated for hours, so you'll feel satisfied longer (remember, your blood glucose level is pivotal to your sense of well-being).

SOURCES OF FAT

Adding fat to a mix of carbohydrates and protein will extend the length of time you'll feel satisfied after eating—up to six hours or more. When adding fats to your meal, try to use unsaturated sources. When eating a more saturated source, try balancing it with unsaturated fat sources in a side dish or at your next meal (depending on the number of calories consumed).

Mostly Unsaturated Fat

most vegetable oils
nuts, seeds
nut butters
avocado
olives
soy products
fish, seafood

About One-third Saturated Fat

beef and other red meats
chicken and turkey
pork
partially hydrogenated margarines and spreads

Mostly Saturated Fat

butter
whole milk, yogurt
cheese
tropical oils (palm, coconut)

Now, when I tell you to eat more fat, don't misunderstand and think that I want you to go out and eat a pound of cheese. That's not the idea. What I'm advocating is that your meals blend the three nutrients in a way that works for you. It doesn't do any good to load up on carbohydrates when you're either going to walk around hungry in two hours or have to hunt down a candy bar.

CARBOHYDRATES

How Many Do You Need?

How many carbohydrates do you need? I wish I could just give you a number and have you adjust your diet accordingly. But it's not that easy. Our needs are unique, because our bodies work differently. Some people metabolize carbohydrates easily and effectively, so a 60 to 70 percent carbohydrate diet works well for them. For others, the maximum number of calories from carbohydrates may be limited to 50 percent or less. Which is why U.S. government has no Recommended Dietary Allowance (RDA) for carbohydrates. But, for purposes of reducing heart disease, the U.S. Dietary Guidelines suggest a target figure of 58 percent of all daily calories from carbohydrates, preferably from fiber-rich complex carbohydrates such as fruits, vegetables, whole grains, and legumes.

As we learn more about the interaction between nutrients and our individual metabolisms, scientists are debating the limitations of a one-size-fits-all diet. Someone who doesn't handle carbohydrates well may function best when consuming 175 to 200 grams of carbohydrates a day. Meanwhile, an athlete who depends on carbohydrates for a significant amount of energy may need to consume 600 grams or more a day. This may explain why some people need only 45 to 50 percent of calories from carbohydrates and others benefit from 70 percent of calories from carbohydrates.

Let me say it again: Carbohydrates as a fuel source are essential to your diet. All digestible carbohydrates contribute to your blood glucose supply. Fewer than 60 grams a day, in just a few days, will almost certainly cause your body to suffer something called ketosis, which is what happens when there is not enough carbohydrate, causing fats to break down incompletely. Ketosis develops in people on fasts or very restricted carbohydrate diets.

The carbohydrates in your diet will be more effective when you personalize your eating regimen and individualize it to fit your lifestyle and unique metabolism. Here's where you need to make decisions about how much carbohydrate you require in your diet. Everyone needs a mix. Not all or none.

My best advice for deciding how many carbohydrates to eat each day is this: experiment. Try the different food plans coming up at the end of this section; they range from 45 to 50 percent to 65 to 70 percent of total calories coming from carbohydrate. Try one plan at a time, staying on that plan for at least a week. Keep track of how you feel on each. Are you content after eating, or are you still searching the cupboard for something to make you feel satisfied? Only when you find the plan that gives you the most pleasure, the most satisfaction, can you identify your own optimum range of carbohydrates.

Sources of Carbohydrates

If you're like most people, you probably think of bread, pasta, rice, or potatoes when someone says carbohydrate. Those starchy foods are of course correct. But you could have answered almost any food in the plant family. In fact, the richest sources of carbohydrates are plant foods: fruits and vegetables, as well as the starchy parts of plants, including roots, stems, leaves, and grains. Beans and legumes, despite being good plant sources of protein, are also mostly carbohydrate.

Milk, yogurt, and related products contain simple carbohydrates in the form of lactose. Some low-fat and nonfat milk products, including yogurt, actually provide more calories from carbohydrate than from protein. Because of how the food is manufactured, there's very little carbohydrate left in most cheese products.

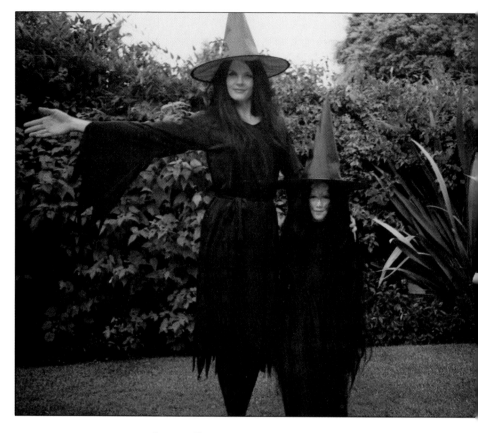

*I love Halloween! Dressing up every year
makes me feel like a kid again.*

All refined sugars and sweeteners are almost 100 percent simple carbohydrate. These include white table sugar, brown sugar, raw sugar, honey, corn syrup, maple syrup, high fructose corn syrup, as well as that well-worn euphemism for sugar—"concentrated fruit juice."

Generally speaking, the less processed the food is, the higher its fiber content and the more likely it is to be considered a complex carbohydrate, even if it contains sugar. The fact is that complex carbohydrates are digested and metabolized more slowly than simple sugars, especially the highly refined sugars, which are very quickly metabolized. Within minutes of consuming simple sugars, blood sugar levels climb—and sometimes plummet just as fast. But when sugars contain significant amounts of fiber (fruits and vegetables, for example), the rate of digestion and absorption of nutrients is greatly slowed. That's why you often feel so much more satisfied over a longer period of time with a piece of fruit as opposed to the equivalent calories in juice.

Absorption and metabolism are also affected by a food particle's size. Compare a bowl of applesauce to a whole apple. They have virtually the same number of grams of carbohydrates and the same calories, but you'd have to chew each bite of the apple about a hundred times to get it down to the same particle size of the applesauce. So the apple is likely to keep you satisfied longer. The smaller the particle size, the faster the digestion, absorption, and metabolism of that particular food.

I've included the following chart in order to show you the range of carbohydrates in our food supply.

CARBOHYDRATES

SERVING SIZE		CARB GRAMS
	BREADS/CEREALS	
4 ounces	plain bagel	61
1 cup	long-grain white rice, cooked	58
1 cup	long-grain brown rice, cooked	45
1 cup	pasta noodles, cooked	38
1 cup	oatmeal cereal, cooked	25
1 cup	Kellogg's Corn Flakes cereal	22
1 each	corn tortilla	14
1 each	pretzels, thick Dutch twist	13
1 piece	cracked wheat bread	12
4 each	saltine crackers	9
	VEGETABLES	
1 cup	sweet potato, peeled	49
1 cup	yellow corn, frozen, boiled	34
1 cup	potato, boiled in skin, peeled	31

SERVING SIZE		CARB GRAMS
1 cup	green peas, frozen	20
1 cup	beets, boiled, diced	17
1 cup	carrots, raw slices	16
1 cup	broccoli pieces, boiled	8
1 cup	cabbage, shredded, raw	4
5 each	asparagus spears, boiled	3
1 cup	romaine lettuce, chopped	1

FRUIT

1 cup	peaches in juice, canned	29
1 each	banana	27
1 cup	fresh fruit salad, no citrus	26
8 ounces	fresh orange juice	24
1 cup	fresh grapefruit juice	23
1 each	medium apple with peel	21
20 each	Thompson seedless grapes	18
1 each	medium orange	16
1 cup	cantaloupe/muskmelon, cubes	13
1 cup	whole strawberries	10

DAIRY

1 cup	low-fat yogurt, fruit	47
1 cup	nonfat yogurt, vanilla/coffee	43
1 cup	nonfat frozen yogurt	38
1 cup	low-fat yogurt, plain	17
1 cup	nonfat skim milk	12
1 cup	2% low-fat milk	12
1 cup	1% low-fat milk	12
1 cup	whole milk	11
1 cup	2% low-fat cottage cheese	8

REFINED SUGARS

1 ounce	hard candy, all flavors	28
1 tablespoon	honey	17
1 tablespoon	light corn syrup	16
1 tablespoon	pancake syrup	15
1 tablespoon	molasses	14
1 tablespoon	jam/preserves	13
1 tablespoon	white granulated sugar	13
1 tablespoon	brown sugar, packed	9
1 tablespoon	reduced-sugar jelly	9
1 tablespoon	Pillsbury Lite pancake syrup	7

SERVING SIZE		CARB GRAMS
	PROTEIN FOODS	
1 cup	garbanzo beans/chickpeas	45
1 cup	pinto beans, dry, boiled	44
1 cup	lentils, dry, boiled	40
2 tablespoons	chunky peanut butter	7
1 cup	tofu (soybean curd, regular)	5
2 tablespoons	dry sunflower seeds	3
1 each	boiled egg, extra large	1
3 ounces	Pacific halibut, steamed	0
3 ounces	beef rump roast	0
3 ounces	skinless chicken breast	0

PROTEIN

On and off for years, Americans have been scolded for eating too much protein. And while yes, it's true, some people probably do eat more than they need, there's plenty of evidence that some people now don't eat enough.

How Much Protein Is Enough

Protein is the one energy nutrient that has earned an RDA—0.8 grams of protein per kilogram of body weight.

You figure the amount of protein you need per day by taking your body weight (in pounds) and dividing by 2.2 (the number of pounds in a kilogram). You then take this number and multiply by 0.8. The answer will be expressed as grams (of protein).

> **Example:** You weigh 140 pounds. Dividing 140 by 2.2 gives you 63.64. Multiplying that by 0.8 makes your daily protein recommendation about 51 grams.

The equation changes a bit when you substantially increase your physical activity—for example, long-distance running and weight lifting. Because we need protein in order to synthesize new cells (to replace the ones that break down during intense activity), you'll have to up your protein intake a bit. So instead of multiplying your weight in kilograms by 0.8, multiply by 1.2 to 1.6, depending on the level of activity.

Below is a table that does some of the math for you. This table gives the daily protein recommendations for a range of body weights at three levels of protein intake. Note that the weights are listed in both pounds and kilograms.

IDENTIFYING YOUR PROTEIN NEEDS

This chart will help you approximate your protein needs.

Step 1: Look up your weight in pounds or kilograms in the two far left-hand columns.

Step 2: Identify your protein needs on the top row. Here's a guide:
   A. Use a factor of **0.8 grams** protein (per kilogram body weight per kg BW) if you are **lightly active or sedentary**.
   B. Use a factor of **1.2 grams** protein (per kilogram body weight) if you are **moderately or very active** (6–12 hours of physical activity per week).
   C. Use a factor of **1.6 grams** protein (per kilogram body weight) if you are **extremely active** (15+ hours of physical activity) or involved with intense weight-bearing activity (i.e., weight training or long-distance running).

Step 3: Find the number of grams of protein recommended for you by identifying the number under the appropriate factor that is positioned across from the weight closest to your weight.

WEIGHT (LBS.)	WEIGHT (KG.)	0.8 G PRO (PER KG BW)	1.2 G PRO (PER KG BW)	1.6 G PRO (PER KG BW)
100	45.5	36	55	73
120	54.5	44	65	87
140	63.6	51	76	102
160	72.7	58	87	116
180	81.8	65	98	131
200	90.9	73	109	145

EXAMPLE: A 140-pound person who is very active could benefit from 76 grams of protein per day.

At the lower end of the recommended protein levels, protein may make up 10 to 15 percent of a day's total calories. This compares well to the 12 percent target that the U.S. Dietary Guidelines recommend. It's not uncommon, however, for Americans to consume 20 to 30 percent of their calories each day from protein. While some studies have linked high-protein diets to cardiovascular disease, obesity, osteoporosis, and other maladies, don't be too quick to cut your portions in half—at least not yet.

No study that I'm aware of has drawn a direct cause-and-effect link between eating too much protein and these risks. Many objections to protein focus on red meat, and most critics are probably more concerned about the amount of fat in red meat than the number of grams of protein in it.

From where do you get protein? Take a look at the next table, which lists several protein-rich foods. As before, the foods are categorized in food groups using standard serving sizes. You'll see that all protein does not come from just meat and dairy products. For a quick assessment, ballpark the number of protein grams in what you ate yesterday. Compare that number to the recommended protein intake on the previous chart. Did you eat enough?

PROTEIN

SERVING SIZE		PROTEIN GRAMS
	BREADS/CEREALS	
4 ounces	plain bagel	12
1 cup	pasta noodles, cooked	6
1 cup	oatmeal cereal, cooked	6
1 cup	long-grain white rice, cooked	6
1 cup	long-grain brown rice, cooked	5
1 piece	cracked wheat bread	2
1 cup	Kellogg's Corn Flakes cereal	2
1 each	corn tortilla	2
1 each	pretzels, thick Dutch twist	1
4 each	saltine crackers	1
	VEGETABLES	
1 cup	green peas, frozen	8
1 cup	yellow corn, frozen, boiled	5
1 cup	broccoli pieces, boiled	5
1 cup	sweet potato, peeled	3
1 cup	potato, boiled in skin, peeled	3
1 cup	beets, boiled, diced	3
5 each	asparagus spears, boiled	2
1 cup	carrots, raw slices	2
1 cup	cabbage, shredded, raw	1
1 cup	romaine lettuce, chopped	1
	FRUIT	
1 each	banana	<1
1 each	medium orange	<1
1 cup	cantaloupe/muskmelon, cubes	<1
1 each	medium apple with peel	<1
1 cup	peaches in juice, canned	<1
1 cup	whole strawberries	<1
8 ounces	fresh orange juice	<1
1 cup	fresh fruit salad, no citrus	<1
1 cup	fresh grapefruit juice	<1
20 each	Thompson seedless grapes	<1
	DAIRY	
1 cup	2% low-fat cottage cheese	31
1 cup	low-fat yogurt, plain	13

SERVING SIZE		PROTEIN GRAMS
1 cup	low-fat yogurt, fruit	11
1 cup	nonfat frozen yogurt	10
1 cup	nonfat skim milk	8
1 cup	2% low-fat milk	8
1 cup	whole milk	8
1 ounce	mozzarella cheese, part-skim	8
1 each	boiled egg, extra large	7
1 ounce	cheddar cheese, diced	7
2 each	egg white, cooked	7
ANIMAL PRODUCTS		
3 ounces	beef rump roast	27
3 ounces	skinless chicken breast	26
3 ounces	chicken breast, roasted	25
3 ounces	salmon fillet, steamed	23
3 ounces	skinless chicken thigh	22
3 ounces	light tuna in water, canned	22
3 ounces	chicken thigh, roasted	21
3 ounces	beef whole rib	19
3 ounces	Pacific halibut, steamed	19
3 ounces	small shrimp, steamed/boiled	18
VEGETABLE PROTEINS		
1 cup	green soybeans, boiled	22
1 cup	tofu (soybean curd, regular)	20
1 cup	lentils, dry, boiled	18
1 cup	split peas, dry, boiled	16
1 cup	garbanzo beans/chickpeas	15
1 cup	pinto beans, dry, boiled	14
2 tablespoons	chunky peanut butter	8
1 cup	split pea soup, dry mix	7
1 ounce	dry roasted cashews	4
2 tablespoons	dry sunflower seeds	4

WHAT KIND OF PROTEIN: Both vegetable and animal sources serve the body well. If you prefer a vegetarian diet, there's no reason why you shouldn't be able to get enough protein. As you can see from the preceding chart, grains and vegetables can add a significant amount of protein to your diet. But if you cut out all animal products, you'll probably need to eat a good amount of beans or legumes each day.

COUNTING PROTEIN CALORIES: Even if you consume enough protein each day, if you don't also consume an adequate number of calories, you're not getting all the bang you can from your protein buck. Why not?

- Protein can be metabolized for energy.
- The body takes care of its energy needs first.
- If you don't consume enough carbohydrates and fat, your body must use protein for fuel.
- If you use protein for energy, your body doesn't have enough of it left to meet its primary need, the growth and development of new cells.
- Growth and development of new cells impacts almost every bodily function; every tissue relies on adequate protein to maintain itself.

So how do you know how many calories are enough? This isn't an easy question to answer. I find that it's best to let hunger and satiety be your guide. Your calorie needs can be extremely variable and depend on many factors that I'll discuss later in the section on metabolism.

FAT

Is there a word today that carries a more sinister connotation? For Americans, fat has become the all-purpose taboo. Foods that have fat are "bad." Nonfat foods are "good." And never the twain shall meet.

"Steak?"

"No, never. Not me. Too much fat."

The major protein sources, gram for gram, differ wildly in their fat contents. Even among different cuts of beef there are huge disparities in fat, while protein content remains relatively consistent. The truth is that every protein source has high- and low-fat choices.

STEAK DINNER COMPARISON

HIGHER FAT OPTION		LOWER FAT OPTION	
Menu	**Fat Grams**	**Menu**	**Fat Grams**
6 ounces Beef Prime Rib	53	6 ounces Beef Top Sirloin Steak	12
1 tablespoon Italian Dressing	7	1 tablespoon Italian Dressing	7
½ tablespoon Butter	6	½ tablespoon Butter	6
2 ounces French Bread	2	2 ounces French Bread	2
1 cup Green Beans	<1	1 cup Green Beans	<1
2 cups Mixed Greens	<1	2 cups Mixed Greens	<1
6 ounces Baked Potato	<1	6 ounces Baked Potato	<1
TOTAL FAT GRAMS	**68 g**	**TOTAL FAT GRAMS**	**27 g**

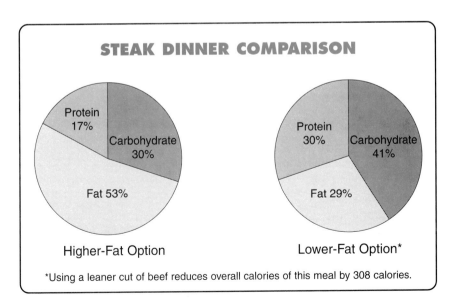

STEAK DINNER COMPARISON

Higher-Fat Option

Protein 17%
Carbohydrate 30%
Fat 53%

Lower-Fat Option*

Protein 30%
Carbohydrate 41%
Fat 29%

*Using a leaner cut of beef reduces overall calories of this meal by 308 calories.

Additional comparisons:

- A piece of trimmed eye of the round contains about 28 per-cent fat, while prime rib has 83 percent (that's one reason why it's so tender and tastes so good).
- Skinless chicken breast provides 23 percent fat, while a wing is loaded with 68 percent—and that's a wing that hasn't been fried or drenched in ranch dressing.
- Turkey breast meat can be as lean as 8 percent fat, compared to standard ground turkey at 58 percent.
- Fish ranges from 10 percent fat in shrimp and tuna to 60 per-cent fat in Atlantic salmon.

*All figures refer to percent of calories from fat, not weight.

Obviously, you can't then argue that *all* red meat is bad or *all* chicken good.

Fat Is an Essential Nutrient

With so many fat-free food products competing for shelf space in the market, it's easy to forget that fat is in fact an essential nutri-ent. Your body absolutely needs it.

How much? Like the other energy nutrients, it depends.

Though fat does not have an RDA assigned to it, the U.S. Dietary Guidelines recommend that no more than 30 percent of your calories come from fat. Some people have found 10 to 15 per-cent of calories from fat just perfect. Others want or need more.

Since fat is the other significant source of energy that your body uses, the amount you require depends on both your total energy needs and how well you metabolize carbohydrates. If you don't handle carbohydrates well, you may need more fat in your diet to provide the energy you need.

To help you determine just how much fat is functional in your diet, let me explain the important functions fat serves in your body and food.

FUNCTIONS OF FAT IN YOUR BODY: If you have a dog, then you've probably bought dog foods that claim to improve the coat and skin. They do that because they contain essential fats—which humans also need to aid growth and maintain good hair and skin. More than that, though, some fats play a powerful role in many body functions, as do other fat-soluble nutrients.

This raises a good point about Americans and their obsession with limiting—even eliminating—fat from their diet. Like carbohydrates, not all fats are created equal. To a large extent, the greatest problem in American diets is an excessive amount of **saturated** fats versus **unsaturated** fats. U.S. Dietary Guidelines recommend limiting saturated fat to less than one-third of your total fat intake.

Look at the chart on the next page. As you can see, most animal sources of protein do not have excessive amounts of saturated fat, with the exceptions, possibly, of whole-milk dairy products, which may contain up to 80 percent saturated fat. And while that high figure doesn't make these products any more taboo than anything else, you do have to be responsible for the amounts of them you eat.

Here are a few important points to remember about fat:

- Unsaturated fat contains essential fatty acids.
- Adequate unsaturated fat is vital to many body functions, even the ability to metabolize carbohydrates and fats.
- Cholesterol is fat soluble. The body needs a certain amount of cholesterol because it's a component of every cell. And it's necessary for the production of important hormones like testosterone, progesterin, and estrogen.
- Essential vitamins A, D, E, and K are fat soluble. While A, D, and K may be synthesized from other sources, vitamin E is the one fat-soluble vitamin we need dietary fat to deliver.

Does all this make it clear that you do not have to get crazy about every little gram of fat you put in your mouth? I hope so.

FAT

SERVING SIZE		FAT GRAMS	SATURATED FAT GRAMS
BREAD/CEREALS			
1 cup	oatmeal cereal	2	
4 ounces	plain bagel	2	
1 cup	long-grain brown rice, cooked	2	
4 each	saltine crackers	1	
1 piece	cracked wheat bread	1	
1 cup	pasta noodles, cooked	1	
1 each	corn tortilla	1	
1 cup	long-grain white rice, cooked	<1	
1 each	pretzels, thick Dutch twist	<1	
1 cup	Kellogg's Corn Flakes cereal	<1	
VEGETABLES			
1 cup	broccoli pieces, boiled	1	
1 cup	green peas, frozen	1	
1 cup	beets, boiled, diced	<1	
1 cup	carrots, raw slices	<1	
5 each	asparagus spears, boiled	<1	
1 cup	sweet potato, peeled	<1	
1 cup	cabbage, shredded, raw	<1	
1 cup	potato, boiled in skin, peeled	<1	
1 cup	yellow corn, frozen, boiled	<1	
1 cup	romaine lettuce, chopped	<1	
FRUIT			
1 cup	fresh fruit salad, no citrus	1	
20 each	Thompson seedless grapes	1	
1 each	banana	1	
1 cup	whole strawberries	1	
1 each	medium apple with peel	<1	
8 ounces	fresh orange juice	<1	
1 cup	cantaloupe/muskmelon, cubes	<1	
1 cup	fresh grapefruit juice	<1	
1 each	medium orange	<1	
1 cup	peaches in juice, canned	<1	

SERVING SIZE		FAT GRAMS	SATURATED FAT GRAMS
DAIRY			
1 ounce	cheddar cheese, diced	9	6
1 cup	whole milk	8	5
1 each	boiled egg, extra large	6	2
1 ounce	mozzarella cheese, part-skim	5	3
1 cup	2% low-fat milk	5	3
1 cup	2% low-fat cottage cheese	4	3
1 cup	low-fat yogurt, plain	4	2
1 cup	low-fat yogurt, fruit	3	2
1 cup	nonfat skim milk	<1	<1
1 cup	nonfat frozen yogurt	<1	<1
2 each	egg white, cooked	0	0
ANIMAL PROTEINS			
3 ounces	beef, prime rib	27	11
3 ounces	chicken thigh, roasted	13	4
3 ounces	skinless chicken thigh	9	3
3 ounces	chicken breast, roasted	7	2
3 ounces	salmon fillet, steamed	6	1
3 ounces	beef rump roast	6	2
3 ounces	skinless chicken breast	3	1
3 ounces	Pacific halibut	3	<1
3 ounces	small shrimp, steamed/boiled	1	<1
3 ounces	light tuna in water, canned	1	<1
VEGETABLE PROTEINS			
2 tablespoons	chunky peanut butter	16	3
1 ounce	dry roasted cashews	13	3
1 cup	tofu (soybean curd, regular)	12	2
1 cup	green soybeans, boiled	12	1
2 tablespoons	dry sunflower seeds	9	1
1 cup	garbanzo beans/chickpeas	4	<1
1 cup	split pea soup, dry mix	1	<1
1 cup	pinto beans, dry, boiled	1	<1
1 cup	split peas, dry, boiled	1	<1
1 cup	lentils, dry, boiled	1	<1

SERVING SIZE		FAT GRAMS	SATURATED FAT GRAMS
ADDED FATS			
1 tablespoon	safflower oil	14	1
1 tablespoon	canola oil	14	1
1 tablespoon	olive oil	14	2
1 tablespoon	lard (pork fat)	13	5
1 tablespoon	butter	12	7
1 tablespoon	Fleischmann's corn oil margarine (stick)	11	2
1 tablespoon	Fleischmann's corn oil margarine (tub)	11	2
1 tablespoon	mayonnaise	11	2
1 tablespoon	blue cheese dressing	8	2
1 tablespoon	Italian dressing	7	1
1 tablespoon	ranch dressing	6	1
1 tablespoon	Shedd's Spread margarine (tub)	6	1
1 tablespoon	cream cheese	5	3
1 tablespoon	Hollandaise sauce	5	3
1 tablespoon	cultured sour cream	3	2
1 tablespoon	low-cal mayonnaise	3	1
1 tablespoon	heavy whipping cream	3	2
1 tablespoon	powdered coffee whitener	2	2
1 tablespoon	half & half cream	2	1
1 tablespoon	nondairy creamer (Mocha Mix)	2	<1
1 tablespoon	guacamole with tomatoes	2	<1
1 tablespoon	beef gravy, homemade	1	<1
1 tablespoon	chicken giblet gravy, homemade	1	<1
1 tablespoon	barbecue sauce	<1	<1

** Saturated fat values are only included for those food groups that contribute significant sources of fat in the diet—dairy, animal proteins, vegetable proteins, and added fats.

THE FUNCTIONS OF FAT IN FOOD: Fat slows digestion. And that's good news.

As I mentioned before, including fat in your diet can help you feel satisfied longer than if there's no fat in your food. Fat can actually improve your weight-management efforts, because the longer you're satisfied, the fewer trips you will have to make to the refrig-

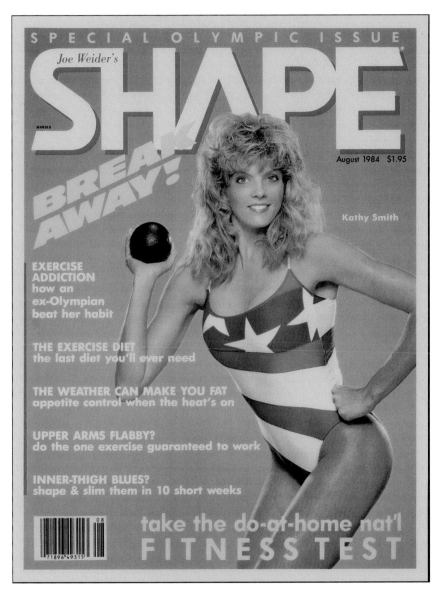

Shape magazine, 1984.

erator or cupboard between meals. (Refer back to the charts in the Food Composition section.)

For example, if you eat a high-carbohydrate meal—maybe a bagel and some fruit salad, or pasta with a light marinara sauce—you'll probably feel hungry within two hours.

Adding some protein to the same food—maybe a bit of nonfat cottage cheese to the bagel, or seafood to the pasta—will slow down digestion enough to keep you feeling satisfied up to four hours.

Now add some fat to the meal—say, a couple of tablespoons of nuts to the fruit salad, or a few meatballs instead of seafood to the pasta—and you'll get the full benefit of balanced eating. You may feel satisfied up to six hours . . . until your next meal.

Then there's the all-important matter of taste. Fat is often the source of food's most intense flavors, so doing away with it leaves your palate searching elsewhere for satisfaction. Example: More than half of mustard's calories come from fat, while chili powder gets almost 60 percent of its calories from fat. Sure, at just a few calories a tablespoon, there's not much risk of putting on weight from too much mustard on your burger. What's important to remember is that mustard's sharp tang, which makes the burger so much better, is due to its fat content. You can't eliminate fat from your diet without missing something. How incredibly bland and boring our food would be without fat.

My opinion is that the biggest problem with fat-free foods is trying to make up for the savoriness that fat provides. Think of the last time you tried a fat-free salad dressing, for example. It didn't roll around your tongue, or have the flavor of oil-based dressings. As for the fat-free desserts, the problem is that the manufacturers try to cover up for the absence of fat by adding too much sugar. The result is often too sweet—and typically not very good.

Truth is, fat in moderation is wonderful. Eat a real cookie, a real brownie, some real dressing. Enjoy your steak, but one that is trimmed and from a lean cut. You may find yourself so happy to enjoy their goodness that you feel satisfied with less.

WATER

Water is that other necessity, besides air, that you can't get along without for very long. Here are a few facts about water:

- Water is a component of every cell in your body.
- Water is the most important and abundant "ingredient" in your body.
- Water comprises 55 to 60 percent of your total body weight.
- You may survive three months without food, but only a few days without water.
- Water carries nutrients from the digestive system to all cells in the body.
- Water carries waste products from the cells to the kidneys so that they can be excreted in urine.
- Water serves as the solution in which all other nutrients are dissolved.
- Water acts as a lubricant and cushion around joints.
- Water serves as a shock absorber inside the eyes and spinal cord.
- Water regulates the body's temperature via sweating, especially during exercise.

Water: How Do You Know How Much Is Enough?

Water comes from two major sources: the fluids you drink and the food you eat.

It's hard to overestimate the importance of water to your good health. Unfortunately, too many people don't make enough of an effort to get all the water they need into their bodies.

You've heard that you're supposed to drink about eight glasses of water a day. I agree with that. But what may surprise you is that all fluids contribute to your fluid intake, not just water. While water is certainly the optimum source of fluids, other liquids such as tea, lemonade, soda, and coffee contribute something to your fluid stores. (Naturally, beverages that have caffeine or alcohol interfere with hydration, since they contain known diuretics, which cause your body to eliminate additional fluids.) Even with a diet rich in water-filled fruits and vegetables, it's a good idea to consume eight glasses of water or other fluids each day.

KATHY'S WATER TIPS

Here's what I've done to get my eight glasses of water a day:

- I drink a glass as soon as I wake up.
- I drink a glass before working out.
- I drink a glass after working out.
- I drink a glass whenever I'm feeling a little low on energy.
- If something hurts (like a headache), I drink a glass.
- If my complexion seems a little dry when I look in the mirror, I drink a glass.
- I always keep a bottle of water at my desk or work area, and next to me in the car.
- I drink out of a twelve-ounce glass instead of an eight-ounce glass, in order to get more throughout the day.
- I drink a glass before dinner.

Still, there's no escaping the truth that if you exercise intensely and work up a good sweat, you probably need to be more conscientious and diligent in order to replace the fluids that your body loses.

Dehydration causes fatigue and contributes to a huge range of symptoms, from poor concentration to headaches, blurred vision, and lack of neuromuscular control. That's not to scare you, only to let you know how important it is to drink freely all the time, not just during and after physical activity.

However, staying hydrated when you're physically active is especially important. To give you an idea why, just once weigh yourself before you start exercising. Then, after you finish, weigh yourself again. Every pound lost during your workout represents sixteen fluid ounces. Naturally, you'll need to replace that fluid in order to stay well-hydrated. It's easy to lose one to three pounds of water weight—or more—every time you exercise.

Remember that thirst is not an adequate measure of how much

water you need. People who sweat heavily will dehydrate faster than their body can signal that they are thirsty. This is especially true for children and the elderly.

PRACTICAL ADVANTAGES OF BEING WELL-HYDRATED

- A greater sense of energy and well-being all the time (after all, water is necessary for every metabolic activity in the body)
- Greater stamina and endurance during physical activity (the body avoids overheating when it can easily sweat)
- Better digestion and elimination (one of the most common causes of constipation is dehydration—even when you get enough fiber!)
- Less chance of overeating (too often people grab something to eat when they actually need something to drink)
- Less chance of holding on to extra water weight. If the body gets a lot of fluids, it will more readily excrete the excess sodium (from last night's dinner) instead of making you feel bloated

---

The Power of Choice Food Plan

How many times have you started a new diet that seems perfect—just what you're looking for—only to find yourself frustrated and ready to give up after a few days? The menus and recipes that looked just great three weeks ago are now giving you fits. You don't like oatmeal and you're supposed to eat it every other day. You don't like the salmon recipe on Day 4, you're not fond of barley, but you're supposed to be eating it for dinner. You happen to love vegetables, but aren't happy to eat fruit three times a day.

Then there is the problem with amounts. You are trying to "be good" but you're hungry! Maybe it's the too small portions, but it could also be not enough fat, maybe not enough carbohydrate, possibly not enough protein. This is not the diet for you after all. You realize you need something more personalized, a way of eating that serves you and your lifestyle. You need the power of choice.

The Power of Choice Food Plan is a unique approach to eating. First, the food plan incorporates everything you have learned about the nutrients and how they can work. And you've learned that some people function best with a high-carbohydrate diet, others function best with more protein and fat. This is why I've developed three eating plans, each designed to address these different needs.

MEAL PLANS: THREE WAYS TO EAT

Meal Plan #1—The Starter

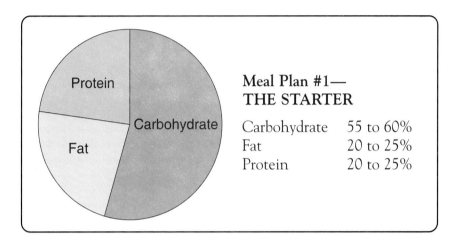

Meal Plan #1—
THE STARTER

Carbohydrate	55 to 60%
Fat	20 to 25%
Protein	20 to 25%

Plan #1 gives you the basic high-carbohydrate low-fat diet. The U.S. Dietary Guidelines and the American Heart Association recommend a similar high-carbohydrate and low-fat diet because most people handle carbohydrates just fine.

Most people will do really well with this food plan. It is estimated that about 75 percent of the population enjoys a metabolism that handles carbohydrates very well. This food plan will give you a nice balance of protein and fat so you can enjoy a wide variety of foods and not be preoccupied with cutting out every possible gram of fat from your diet.

Meal Plan #2–The Carbo-Loader

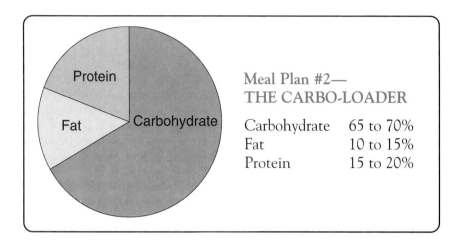

Meal Plan #2—
THE CARBO-LOADER

Carbohydrate	65 to 70%
Fat	10 to 15%
Protein	15 to 20%

Plan #2 is higher in carbohydrate and lower in fat. If you are extremely active, or really enjoy carbohydrates and they work well for you and you actually enjoy eating very little fat, you may find yourself best suited for Plan 2. Vegetarians who choose a low-fat diet will typically find themselves eating a similar ratio of carbohydrates and fats.

Meal Plan #3–The Hunter-Gatherer

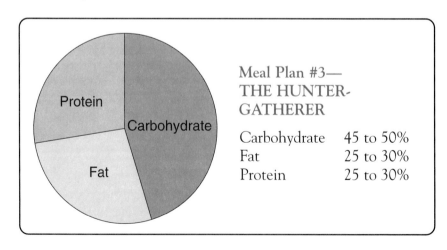

Meal Plan #3—
THE HUNTER-
GATHERER

Carbohydrate	45 to 50%
Fat	25 to 30%
Protein	25 to 30%

Plan #3 is designed for those individuals who do better with more protein and fat in their diet. People who don't handle carbohydrates well are thought to be relatively insulin resistant. Insulin resistance or carbohydrate sensitivity is basically a glitch in the body's ability to effectively metabolize carbohydrates. Scientists have found that there is a huge range of insulin resistance among people for a lot of different reasons.

The most common reason people develop insulin resistance is because they gain fat weight. Insulin resistance is twice as common in obese individuals than those with less body fat.

Another critical factor is physical activity. Too little physical activity contributes to insulin resistance for two reasons. Physical activity enhances the ability for your body to metabolize carbohydrates effectively. This benefit is lost after sixty hours following your last exercise session. In addition, without physical activity your metabolism will slow down. Once we finish growing and developing—at about twenty-five years of age—muscle mass will atrophy unless we do something to maintain it or build it up. Muscle mass is one of the factors that can increase your metabolic rate that you get to control. A strong metabolic rate means you can eat more, feel more satisfied, and be less likely to gain fat weight.

Diet plays the next most significant role. Since insulin resistance is about carbohydrate metabolism, the amount of carbohydrate in your diet may be the difference between gaining weight and losing weight, as well as the difference between a great sense of well-being and feeling sluggish and fatigued. It is really the difference between your body's cells getting to metabolize nutrients effectively for energy or storing this energy as fat.

Currently, science doesn't have easy ways to determine how much carbohydrate we can handle, nor is it easy to test for insulin resistance. This is especially true the younger you are. You may be born with a predisposition to be insulin resistant. But that predisposition may never be realized or not be evident until you are much older, more out of shape, and/or carry more body fat.

Even so, those individuals who are predisposed to insulin resistance may find that eating more protein and fat, with less carbohydrate, is a much more functional way to eat. This mix of nutrients just works for you better in every way. You may notice:

- you feel less hungry after a meal and satisfied longer
- you don't crave sugars and carbohydrates as much
- you feel satisfied even eating fewer calories than before
- you feel more alert and energized all day long
- you don't get as many or as severe "hypoglycemic" symptoms such as dizziness, shakiness, inability to concentrate, or headaches
- you lose fat weight more readily, especially if you carry it in your abdominal area or more in your torso than your arms and legs
- you feel stronger and don't feel so weak when you exercise or after you exercise
- you feel less bloated and thick in your torso

Despite the fact that you will be eating a lower amount of carbohydrate, "The Hunter-Gatherer" is still very moderate in fat. Most recommendations for a lower-fat diet specify that fat intake should be equal to or less than 30 percent from total calories. With this plan you get the benefit of eating a balance of carbohydrate, protein, and fat that works for you and still enjoy the fact that you are eating a healthful diet.

PUTTING IT ALL TOGETHER

After reading this, you may be wondering how you can possibly make sense of everything. That's why I've done it for you, putting together meal plans you can refer to easily and quickly—plans that are flexible and offer you different food compositions, so you can determine which works best for you. Really, all you have to do is observe yourself and see how you respond to the three different plans in order to come to a much easier and more functional relationship with food. Each meal plan contains ten breakfast and twenty lunch/dinner options with a calorie-per-meal range of 450 to 550. I've color coded the three plans to make it easier for you to follow (Meal Plan #1—The Starter in blue, Meal Plan #2—The Carbo-Loader in green, and Meal Plan #3—The Hunter-Gatherer in red). If you require more calories, feel free to eat more of each item or include your favorite snacks. Also, note that lunch and dinner are interchangeable.

It's probably not wise for most active women to eat fewer than 1,500 calories a day—even when trying to lose fat weight. So many factors determine your real metabolic needs that no basic food plan can satisfy everyone perfectly. That's why you should base your own calorie intake on your level of hunger. The key is to stop when you've had enough. For men, the daily minimum number of calories may be 1,800, more or less.

You may have noticed that I have presented each of the food plans with ranges of each nutrient (i.e., 55 to 60 percent calories from carbohydrate). This allows me to present food plans that contain more flexible food choices. It goes without saying, though, that these are not the only meal plans that could work for you.

Meal Plan #1—THE STARTER

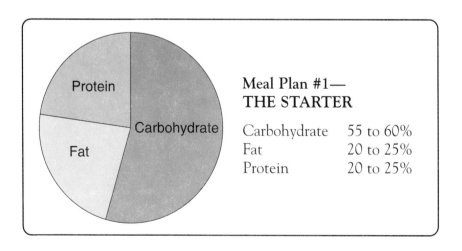

**Meal Plan #1—
THE STARTER**

Carbohydrate	55 to 60%
Fat	20 to 25%
Protein	20 to 25%

Breakfast Options

Oatmeal Blueberry Pancake Breakfast

3 each   Oatmeal Blueberry Pancakes (recipe p. 143) with 2 tablespoons Maple Syrup

2 ounces   Whole Ham, roasted and trimmed

1 cup   Fresh Berries

Calories	489
Nutrient Breakdown	
• Protein	24 grams
• Carbohydrates	76 grams
• Fat	12 grams
Saturated Fat	3 grams

Recipe Tip:
You can easily substitute any berry, apples, or bananas in the pancake recipe. Also, you may substitute Canadian bacon, a lean hamburger patty, or minute steak.

Breakfast Quesadilla and Melon

4 each   Corn Tortillas

¾ ounce   Part-Skim, Low-Moisture Mozzarella Cheese, shredded

1 ounce weight   Skinless Chicken Breast, roasted

2 tablespoons   Salsa

1 cup   Cantaloupe/Muskmelon, cubed

Calories	487
Nutrient Breakdown	
• Protein	28 grams
• Carbohydrates	73 grams
• Fat	11 grams
Saturated Fat	5 grams

Recipe Tip:
If you prefer flour tortillas substitute 1 10-inch flour tortilla for every 2 corn tortillas.

Apple Brunch Breakfast

4 ounces	Apple Brunch Corn Cakes (recipe p. 144)
6 ounces	2% Low-Fat Cottage Cheese
1 cup	Fresh Fruit Salad
1 teaspoon	Butter

Calories	484
Nutrient Breakdown	
• Protein	29 grams
• Carbohydrates	67 grams
• Fat	13 grams
Saturated Fat	5 grams

Recipe Tip:
Anytime fresh fruit salad is included in a menu plan you can substitute 1 cup of any cut-up fresh fruit.

Cold Cereal Breakfast

1½ cups	Shredded Wheat Cereal, small biscuit
1 cup	2% Lower-Fat Milk
1 cup	Whole Strawberries
2 tablespoons	Dried Black Walnuts

Calories	489
Nutrient Breakdown	
• Protein	20 grams
• Carbohydrates	75 grams
• Fat	16 grams
Saturated Fat	4 grams

Recipe Tip:
Substitute any cold cereal:
• 1 ½ cups shredded wheat is equivalent to 2 ¼ ounces other cold cereals.

Bagel and Lox Breakfast

3 ounces	Plain Bagel
3 tablespoons	Low-Fat Cream Cheese
2 ounces	Smoked Chinook Salmon/Lox
1 cup	Fresh Fruit Salad

Calories	**505**
Nutrient Breakdown	
• Protein	25 grams
• Carbohydrates	74 grams
• Fat	12 grams
Saturated Fat	6 grams

Recipe Tip:
Instead of salmon lox enjoy other smoked fish or lean deli meats. They work just as well and offer more variety.

Peanut Butter Toast Breakfast

2 slices	Cracked Wheat Bread
2 tablespoons	Chunky Peanut Butter
2 cups	Fresh Fruit Salad

Calories	**520**
Nutrient Breakdown	
• Protein	14 grams
• Carbohydrates	83 grams
• Fat	19 grams
Saturated Fat	4 grams

Recipe Tip:
Using peanut butter in a meal means your fat content will be higher than usual. Because the fats in nuts and seeds are primarily unsaturated, any nut butter will work here. Enjoy the convenience!

Oatmeal Breakfast

1½ cups	Oatmeal Cereal, cooked
1 cup	Low-Fat Yogurt, plain
1 tablespoon	Dried Black Walnuts
1 each	Banana

Calories	525
Nutrient Breakdown	
• Protein	25 grams
• Carbohydrates	83 grams
• Fat	12 grams
Saturated Fat	4 grams

Recipe Tip:
Use any favorite dried fruit in your oatmeal. For a heartier consistency try using steel-cut oats.

Eggs and Toast

2 each	Whole Eggs, scrambled with
2 each	Egg Whites
2 slices	Cracked Wheat Bread
1½ cups	Fresh Fruit Salad
½ tablespoon	Jam

Calories	519
Nutrient Breakdown	
• Protein	28 grams
• Carbohydrates	72 grams
• Fat	15 grams
Saturated Fat	4 grams

Recipe Tip:
Any type of bread can be used in this meal (i.e., sourdough, whole grain, rye, oatmeal, pumpernickel). English muffins work well, too.

Waffles and Fruit

2 each	Waffles, frozen or toasted
1 cup	Fresh Strawberries
3 ounces	Whole Ham, roasted and trimmed
2 tablespoons	Maple Syrup

Calories	473
Nutrient Breakdown	
• Protein	27 grams
• Carbohydrates	67 grams
• Fat	11 grams
Saturated Fat	3 grams

Recipe Tip:
Waffles made at home or ordered from a restaurant are larger than typical frozen waffles. You'll probably need to moderate your portion.

French Toast

2 slices	Cracked Wheat Bread
3 each	Raw Whole Egg Whites, extra large
¼ teaspoon	Corn Oil (for cooking)
1 ounce	Ham Dinner Steak, water added
1½ cups	Fresh Fruit Salad
½ tablespoon	Maple Syrup

Calories	469
Nutrient Breakdown	
• Protein	25 grams
• Carbohydrates	72 grams
• Fat	11 grams
Saturated Fat	3 grams

Recipe Tip:
Enhance with a variety of bread. One day use whole wheat, other days sourdough or French. For special occasions, cinnamon-raisin bread.

Lunch and Dinner Options

BBQ Chicken on a Bun

1 each	Mixed Grain Hamburger/Hot Dog Bun
3 ounces	Skinless Chicken Breast, roasted
2 tablespoons	Barbecue Sauce
10 each	Baby Carrots, raw with
2 teaspoons	Ranch Salad Dressing
1½ cups	Fresh Fruit Salad

Calories	503
Nutrient Breakdown	
• Protein	34 grams
• Carbohydrates	70 grams
• Fat	11 grams
Saturated Fat	2 grams

Recipe Tip:
Lean roast beef and pork tenderloin also work well in this sandwich. Be sure to not overcook the pork. The pork is done when juices run clear.

Curried Chicken-Cilantro Salad

6 ounces	Curried Chicken-Cilantro Salad (recipe p. 146)
2 ounces	Hard White Roll
1 cup	Fresh Fruit Salad

Calories	468
Nutrient Breakdown	
• Protein	26 grams
• Carbohydrates	65 grams
• Fat	13 grams
Saturated Fat	2 grams

Recipe Tip:
For an easy on-the-go meal try stuffing the chicken cilantro salad into a pita or rolling it into a tortilla or a piece of lavosh bread.

❧✻❧✻❧✻

Zesty Low-Fat Spinach Salad

1 each	Zesty Spinach Salad (recipe p. 147)
3 ounces	Honey Roast Turkey Breast
½ cup	Fresh Fruit Salad

Calories	**511**	
Nutrient Breakdown		
• Protein	23 grams	
• Carbohydrates	75 grams	
• Fat	17 grams	
Saturated Fat	3 grams	

Recipe Tip:
Other grain options include bulgur, couscous, or a mix of brown and wild rice. Remember, brown rice takes a bit longer to cook than other grains.

❧✻❧✻❧✻

Grilled Hamburger

3 ounces	Beef Round-Eye (choice)
1 each	Hamburger Bun
2 leaves	Iceberg/Crisphead Lettuce
2 slices	Fresh Tomato
1 slice	Red Onion
1 tablespoon	Prepared Mustard
1 tablespoon	Low-Calorie Mayonnaise
5 slices	Dill Pickle
1¾ cups	Fresh Fruit Salad

Calories	**527**	
Nutrient Breakdown		
• Protein	32 grams	
• Carbohydrates	76 grams	
• Fat	12 grams	
Saturated Fat	3 grams	

Recipe Tip:
The leanest ground beef (7% fat by weight) may not hold together well, so try adding an egg white to the raw meat before shaping it into patties.

Steak Lovers' Salad

2 ounces	Beef Tenderloin Steak, broiled
4 cups	Mixed Salad Greens/Lettuce
½ ounce	Honey Dijon Dressing (recipe p.158)
3 ounces	Sourdough Roll
2 cups	Whole Strawberries

Calories	**510**
Nutrient Breakdown	
• Protein	29 grams
• Carbohydrates	75 grams
• Fat	11 grams
Saturated Fat	3 grams

Recipe Tip:
This is a great way to enjoy left-over grilled steak. Of course, grilled chicken or pork can work equally well.

Veggie Pita Pizza

2 each	Whole-Wheat Pita Pocket Bread
½ cup	Tomato Sauce, canned
¼ cup	Sweet Green Bell Peppers, raw, chopped
¼ cup	Onions, raw, chopped
¼ cup	Mushroom Pieces, raw
¼ cup	Part-Skim, Low-Moisture Mozzarella Cheese, shredded
2 cups	Tossed Green Salad
5 slices	Cucumber with Peel
¼ cup	Tomato, chopped
1 tablespoon	Low-Calorie Dressing, oil-free

Calories	520
Nutrient Breakdown	
• Protein	30 grams
• Carbohydrates	78 grams
• Fat	14 grams
Saturated Fat	7 grams

Recipe Tip:
Many other breads work well in this recipe. Boboli, sliced French bread, and sourdough rolls are good options.

Tuna Tostada Meal

1 each	Light and Healthy Tuna Tostada (recipe p. 149)
15 pieces	Baked Tortilla Chips
1 cup	Fresh Fruit Salad

Calories	495
Nutrient Breakdown	
• Protein	32 grams
• Carbohydrates	72 grams
• Fat	11 grams
Saturated Fat	2 grams

Recipe Tip:
For an exotic touch, try using crab, shrimp, squid, or lobster. These are equally low-fat protein sources.

Speedy Salad Burritos

¾ cup	Refried Beans, canned
2 each	Whole-Wheat Tortillas
¼ cup	Cheddar Cheese, shredded
1 cup	Iceberg/Crisphead Lettuce, chopped
¼ cup	Ortega Dipping Salsa

Calories	491
Nutrient Breakdown	
• Protein	25 grams
• Carbohydrates	81 grams
• Fat	12 grams
Saturated Fat	7 grams

Recipe Tip:
Refried beans aren't the high-fat product most assume. One national brand is only 9% calories from fat. Refried black beans can also be used.

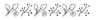

Oriental Turkey Express

4 ounces	Oven Roast Turkey Breast
2 teaspoons	Sesame Oil
¼ cup	Szechwan Sauce
1¼ cups	Japanese Stir-Fry Vegetables
¾ cup	Long-Grain White Rice, cooked

Calories	510
Nutrient Breakdown	
• Protein	32 grams
• Carbohydrates	70 grams
• Fat	13 grams
Saturated Fat	2 gram

Recipe Tip:
You can use a variety of Asian seasonings to enhance this dish. Hoisan sauce will give it a sweeter flavor while a black bean sauce is a very savory option.

Soup and Sandwich

8 ounces	Lentil Soup
2 slices	Cracked Wheat Bread
2 ounces	Beef Round-Eye (choice), trimmed
1 cup	Fresh Fruit Salad
½ tablespoon	Mayonnaise

Calories	500
Nutrient Breakdown	
• Protein	29 grams
• Carbohydrates	70 grams
• Fat	12 grams
Saturated Fat	3 grams

Recipe Tip:
This combination has endless possibilities. Any hearty soup will complement the sandwich nicely. This sandwich can be equally versatile. Try using sliced ham, turkey, or tuna salad.

Mediterranean Pasta Salad

1 cup	Rotini Pasta Noodles, cooked
¾ cup	Garbanzo Beans/Chickpeas, boiled
3 tablespoons	Feta Cheese
2 ounces	Squid (Philippine), boiled
¼ cup	Sweet Raw Green Bell Peppers, chopped
¼ cup	Deluxe Artichoke Hearts
¼ cup	Tomato, chopped
¼ cup	Raw Celery, chopped
¼ cup	Low-Calorie Salad Dressing, oil-free
1 tablespoon	Fresh Lemon Juice

Calories	514
Nutrient Breakdown	
• Protein	30 grams
• Carbohydrates	71 grams
• Fat	13 grams
Saturated Fat	7 grams

Recipe Tip:
The sharp flavor of cheese is a great taste enhancer. Try using Parmesan, Romano, or Gorgonzola for an equally tantalizing flavor.

South-of-the-Border Chili

8 ounces	South-of-the-Border Vegetarian Chili (recipe p. 150)
1½ ounces	Beef Rump Roast, braised and trimmed
2 tablespoons	Cheddar Cheese, shredded
2 medium slices	French Bread
2 cups	Mixed Salad Greens/Lettuce
1 tablespoon	Low-Calorie Dressing, oil-free

Calories	489
Nutrient Breakdown	
• Protein	34 grams
• Carbohydrates	67 grams
• Fat	11 grams
Saturated Fat	5 grams

Recipe Tip:
If you're not a beef lover, you can easily use ground turkey in this recipe.

Seafood Pizza

2 slices	Seafood Pizza (recipe p. 153)
2 cups	Tossed Green Salad
½ each	Medium Whole Tomato
5 slices	Cucumber with Peel
2 tablespoons	Fat-Free Italian Dressing

Calories	496
Nutrient Breakdown	
• Protein	24 grams
• Carbohydrates	72 grams
• Fat	13 grams
Saturated Fat	4 grams

Recipe Tip:
Are you a traditionalist? A great low-fat pizza topping is Canadian bacon. Made from pork tenderloin, it has the same fat content as skinless chicken breast.

Poached Salmon with Mustard-Ginger Sauce

3 ounces	Poached Salmon with Mustard-Ginger Sauce (recipe p. 151)
6 ounces	Roasted Potato
1 teaspoon	Olive Oil
1 cup	Deluxe Sugar Snap Peas

Calories	**520**
Nutrient Breakdown	
• Protein	29 grams
• Carbohydrates	73 grams
• Fat	13 grams
Saturated Fat	2 grams

Recipe Tip:
For a great summer treat, try substituting corn on the cob for the roasted potatoes.

Flank Steak Dinner

3 ounces	Beef Flank Steak (choice), broiled
6 ounces	Garlicky Mashed Potatoes (recipe p. 148)
2 cups	Mixed Salad Greens/Lettuce
2 tablespoons	Fat-Free Italian Dressing
2 medium slices	French Bread

Calories	**517**
Nutrient Breakdown	
• Protein	33 grams
• Carbohydrates	70 grams
• Fat	11 grams
Saturated Fat	4 grams

Recipe Tip:
Flank is not the only lean meat great on the grill or broiled. Other options include: top sirloin, London broil, filet mignon, or beef tenderloin.

Dijon Parmesan Halibut

3 ounces	Dijon Parmesan Halibut (recipe p. 157)
1¼ cups	Long-Grain Brown Rice, cooked and hot
1 cup	Broccoli Pieces, boiled
2 cups	Mixed Salad Greens/Lettuce
2 tablespoons	Low-Calorie Italian Dressing
1 tablespoon	Parmesan Cheese, grated

Calories	**496**
Nutrient Breakdown	
• Protein	31 grams
• Carbohydrates	71 grams
• Fat	11 grams
Saturated Fat	3 grams

Recipe Tip:
Any firm-fleshed fish will do: try swordfish, sea bass, or orange roughy.

Broccoli Tofu Stir-Fry

8 ounces	Broccoli Tofu Stir-Fry (recipe p. 154)
1½ cups	Long-Grain Rice, cooked

Calories	**492**
Nutrient Breakdown	
• Protein	26 grams
• Carbohydrates	73 grams
• Fat	11 grams
Saturated Fat	1 gram

Recipe Tip:
Any lean protein can be substituted for the tofu: lean sirloin beef, trimmed pork tenderloin, skinless chicken, or turkey.

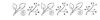

Spicy Oven-Fried Chicken

4 ounces	Spicy Oven-Fried Chicken (recipe p. 152)
6 ounces	Sweet Potato, peeled after baking
1 cup	Green Snap/String Beans, raw or boiled
1 teaspoon	Butter

Calories	505
Nutrient Breakdown	
• Protein	33 grams
• Carbohydrates	69 grams
• Fat	12 grams
Saturated Fat	4 grams

Recipe Tip:
Do you prefer dark meat? Try skinless drumsticks. They contain a mere 28% calories from fat while skinless thighs yield 47% calories from fat.

Pasta Primavera

1 cup	Rotini Pasta Noodles, cooked
2 tablespoons	Garbanzo Beans, dry or boiled
2 tablespoons	Red Kidney Beans, dry or boiled
½ cup	Italian Green Beans, frozen or boiled
¼ cup	Zucchini Squash, boiled
¼ cup	Tomato, chopped
½ cup	Spaghetti with Marinara Sauce
4 tablespoons	Parmesan Cheese, grated

Calories	502
Nutrient Breakdown	
• Protein	25 grams
• Carbohydrates	73 grams
• Fat	14 grams
Saturated Fat	6 grams

Recipe Tip:
Enjoy any mix of vegetables. A variety of green, yellow, and red bell peppers is another great combination.

Black Bean Soup

16 ounces	Black Bean Soup (recipe p. 155)
1 tablespoon	Asiago or Parmesan Cheese, shredded
1 ounce	Mixed Grain Bread
2 cups	Mixed Salad Greens/Lettuce
1 tablespoon	Low-Calorie Italian Dressing
1 cup	Cantaloupe/Muskmelon, cubed

Calories	**508**
Nutrient Breakdown	
• Protein	31 grams
• Carbohydrates	77 grams
• Fat	11 grams
Saturated Fat	5 grams

Recipe Tip:
Any bean, lentil, or split pea soup will work in this meal plan.

Meal Plan #2—THE CARBO-LOADER

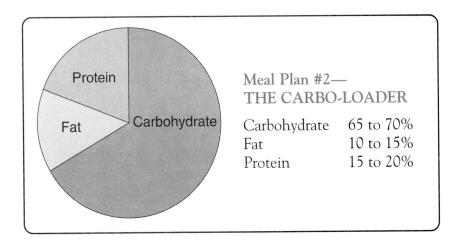

Meal Plan #2—
THE CARBO-LOADER

Carbohydrate	65 to 70%
Fat	10 to 15%
Protein	15 to 20%

Breakfast Options

❧❀❧❀❧❀

Oatmeal Blueberry Pancake Breakfast

2 each	Oatmeal Blueberry Pancakes (recipe p. 143) with 2 tablespoons Maple Syrup
8 ounces	Low-Fat Vanilla Yogurt
½ cup	Fresh Berries (on top of yogurt or on the side)

Calories	481
Nutrient Breakdown	
• Protein	18 grams
• Carbohydrates	88 grams
• Fat	8 grams
Saturated Fat	3 grams

Recipe Tip:
You can easily substitute any berry, apples, or bananas in the pancake recipe.

❧❀❧❀❧❀

Breakfast Quesadilla and Melon

4 each	Corn Tortillas
2 ounces	Low-Sodium, Low-Fat Cheddar Cheese, diced
4 tablespoons	Salsa
1 cup	Cantaloupe/Muskmelon, cubed

Calories	440
Nutrient Breakdown	
• Protein	22 grams
• Carbohydrates	75 grams
• Fat	7 grams
Saturated Fat	3 grams

Recipe Tip:
If you prefer flour tortillas substitute 1 10-inch flour tortilla for every 2 corn tortillas.

Apple Brunch Breakfast

4 ounces	Apple Brunch Corn Cakes (recipe p. 144)
4 ounces	Nonfat Cottage Cheese
2 cups	Fresh Fruit Salad

Calories	469
Nutrient Breakdown	
• Protein	22 grams
• Carbohydrates	89 grams
• Fat	6 grams
Saturated Fat	1 gram

Recipe Tip:
Anytime fresh fruit salad is included in a menu plan you can substitute 1 cup of any cut-up fresh fruit.

Cold Cereal Breakfast

2 cups	Shredded Wheat Cereal
1 cup	2% Low-Fat Milk
1 cup	Whole Strawberries

Calories	471
Nutrient Breakdown	
• Protein	18 grams
• Carbohydrates	90 grams
• Fat	7 grams
Saturated Fat	3 grams

Recipe Tip:
substitute any cold cereal:
· 2 cups shredded wheat is equivalent to 3 ounces of other cold cereals.

Bagel and Lox Breakfast

3 ounces	Plain Bagel
2 tablespoons	Low-Fat Cream Cheese
1 ounce	Smoked Chinook Salmon/Lox
1½ cups	Fresh Fruit Salad

Calories	488
Nutrient Breakdown	
• Protein	19 grams
• Carbohydrates	86 grams
• Fat	9 grams
Saturated Fat	4 grams

Recipe Tip:
Instead of salmon lox enjoy other smoked fish or lean deli meats. They work just as well and offer more variety.

Peanut Butter Toast Breakfast

3 slices	Cracked Wheat Bread
1 tablespoon	Chunky Peanut Butter
2 cups	Fresh Fruit Salad

Calories	491
Nutrient Breakdown	
• Protein	13 grams
• Carbohydrates	92 grams
• Fat	12 grams
Saturated Fat	2 grams

Recipe Tip:
Using peanut butter in a meal means your fat content will be higher than usual. Because the fats in nuts and seeds are primarily unsaturated, any nut butter will work here. Enjoy the convenience!

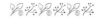

Oatmeal Breakfast

1½ cups	Oatmeal Cereal, cooked
1 cup	2% Lower-Fat Milk
1 tablespoon	Seedless Raisins, packed
1 each	Banana

Calories 474
Nutrient Breakdown
- Protein 19 grams
- Carbohydrates 85 grams
- Fat 9 grams
  Saturated Fat 4 grams

Recipe Tip:
Use any favorite dried fruit in your oatmeal. For a heartier consistency try using steel-cut oats.

Eggs and Toast

4 each	Egg Whites, cooked
2 slices	Cracked Wheat Bread
2 cups	Fresh Fruit Salad
1 teaspoon	Margarine
1 tablespoon	Jam/Preservatives

Calories 481
Nutrient Breakdown
- Protein 20 grams
- Carbohydrates 90 grams
- Fat 7 grams
  Saturated Fat 1 gram

Recipe Tip:
Any type of bread can be used in this meal (i.e., sourdough, whole grain, rye, oatmeal, pumpernickel). English muffins work well, too.

Waffles and Fruit

2 each	Waffles, frozen or toasted
½ cup	Fresh Strawberries, sliced
1 cup	Low-Fat Vanilla Yogurt
2 tablespoons	Maple Syrup

Calories	524
Nutrient Breakdown	
• Protein	17 grams
• Carbohydrates	95 grams
• Fat	9 grams
Saturated Fat	3 grams

Recipe Tip:
Waffles made at home or ordered from a restaurant are larger than typical frozen waffles. You'll probably need to moderate your portion.

French Toast

3 slices	Cracked Wheat Bread
4 each	Raw Egg Whites
¼ teaspoon	Corn Oil (for cooking)
1½ cups	Fresh Fruit Salad
1 tablespoon	Maple Syrup

Calories	479
Nutrient Breakdown	
• Protein	22 grams
• Carbohydrates	92 grams
• Fat	5 grams
Saturated Fat	1 gram

Recipe Tip:
Enhance with a variety of bread. One day use whole wheat, other days sourdough or French. For special occasions, cinnamon-raisin bread.

Lunch and Dinner Options

BBQ Chicken on a Bun

1 each	Mixed Grain Hamburger/Hot Dog Bun
2 ounces	Skinless Chicken Breast, roasted
2 tablespoons	Barbecue Sauce
10 each	Baby Carrots, raw 2.75 inch
2 cups	Fresh Fruit Salad

Calories	**470**
Nutrient Breakdown	
• Protein	25 grams
• Carbohydrates	83 grams
• Fat	7 grams
Saturated Fat	2 grams

Recipe Tip:
Lean roast beef and pork tenderloin also work well in this sandwich. Be sure to not overcook the pork. The pork is done when juices run clear.

Oriental Turkey Express

2½ ounces	Oven Roast Turkey Breast
½ teaspoon	Sesame Oil
¼ cup	Szechwan Sauce
1½ cups	Japanese Stir-Fry Vegetables
1 cup	Long-Grain Rice, cooked

Calories	**495**
Nutrient Breakdown	
• Protein	26 grams
• Carbohydrates	88 grams
• Fat	5 grams
Saturated Fat	1 gram

Recipe Tip:
You can use a variety of Asian seasonings to enhance this dish. Hoisan sauce will give it a sweeter flavor while a black bean sauce is a very savory option.

Soup and Sandwich

12 ounces	Lentil Soup
2 slices	Cracked Wheat Bread
1 ounce	Beef Round-Eye (choice), trimmed
1½ cups	Fresh Fruit Salad

Calories 511
Nutrient Breakdown
• Protein 25 grams
• Carbohydrates 92 grams
• Fat 6 grams
Saturated Fat 1 gram

Recipe Tip:
This combination has endless possibilities. Any hearty soup will complement the sandwich nicely. This sandwich can be equally versatile. Try using sliced ham, turkey, or tuna salad.

Speedy Salad Burritos

1 cup	Refried Beans, canned
2 each	Whole-Wheat Tortillas
2 tablespoons	Part-Skim, Low-Moisture Mozzarella Cheese, shredded
1 cup	Iceberg/Crisphead Lettuce, chopped
¼ cup	Salsa

Calories 484
Nutrient Breakdown
• Protein 26 grams
• Carbohydrates 92 grams
• Fat 6 grams
Saturated Fat 3 grams

Recipe Tip:
Refried beans aren't the high-fat product most assume. One national brand is only 9% calories from fat. Refried black beans can also be used.

Tuna Tostada Meal

1 each	Light and Healthy Tuna Tostada (recipe p. 149)
8 pieces	Baked Tortilla Chips
2 cups	Fresh Fruit Salad

Calories	**524**
Nutrient Breakdown	
• Protein	33 grams
• Carbohydrates	93 grams
• Fat	5 grams
Saturated Fat	1 gram

Recipe Tip:
For an exotic touch, try using crab, shrimp, squid, or lobster. These are equally low-fat protein sources.

Grilled Hamburger

2 ounces	Beef Round-Eye (choice)
1 each	Hamburger Bun
2 leaves	Iceberg/Crisphead Lettuce
2 slices	Fresh Tomato
1 slice	Red Onion
1 tablespoon	Prepared Mustard
5 slices	Dill Pickle
2 cups	Fresh Fruit Salad

Calories	**466**
Nutrient Breakdown	
• Protein	24 grams
• Carbohydrates	80 grams
• Fat	8 grams
Saturated Fat	2 grams

Recipe Tip:
The leanest ground beef (7% fat by weight) may not hold together well, so try adding an egg white to the raw meat before shaping it into patties.

Steak Lovers' Salad

1 ounce	Beef Tenderloin Steak, broiled
4 cups	Mixed Salad Greens/Lettuce
1 ounce	Fat-Free Honey Dijon Dressing
3 ounces	Sourdough Roll
2 cups	Whole Strawberries

Calories	474
Nutrient Breakdown	
• Protein	21 grams
• Carbohydrates	84 grams
• Fat	7 grams
Saturated Fat	2 grams

Recipe Tip:
This is a great way to enjoy leftover grilled steak. Of course, grilled chicken or pork can work equally well.

Veggie Pita Pizza

2 each	Whole-Wheat Pita Pocket Bread
½ cup	Tomato Sauce, canned
¼ cup	Sweet Green Bell Peppers, raw, chopped
¼ cup	Onions, raw, chopped
¼ cup	Mushroom Pieces, raw
¼ cup	Part-Skim, Low-Moisture Mozzarella Cheese, shredded
2 cups	Tossed Green Salad
5 slices	Cucumber with Peel
¼ cup	Tomato, chopped
1 tablespoon	Low-Calorie Dressing, oil-free

Calories	441
Nutrient Breakdown	
• Protein	22 grams
• Carbohydrates	77 grams
• Fat	9 grams
Saturated Fat	4 grams

Recipe Tip:
Many other breads work well in this recipe. Boboli, sliced French bread, and sourdough rolls are good options.

Curried Chicken-Cilantro Salad

3 ounces	Curried Chicken-Cilantro Salad (recipe p. 146)
2 ounces	Hard White Roll
2 cups	Fresh Fruit Salad

Calories	511
Nutrient Breakdown	
• Protein	19 grams
• Carbohydrates	93 grams
• Fat	9 grams
Saturated Fat	2 grams

Recipe Tip:
For an easy on-the-go meal try stuffing the chicken-cilantro salad into a pita or rolling it into a tortilla or a piece of lavosh bread.

Zesty Low-Fat Spinach Salad

1 each	Zesty Spinach Salad (recipe p. 147)
4 each	Egg Whites (cooked)
1 cup	Fresh Fruit Salad

Calories	464
Nutrient Breakdown	
• Protein	21 grams
• Carbohydrates	86 grams
• Fat	7 grams
Saturated Fat	1 gram

Recipe Tip:
Other grain options include bulgur, couscous, or a mix of brown and wild rice. Remember, brown rice takes a bit longer to cook than other grains.

Mediterranean Pasta Salad

1 cup	Rotini Pasta Noodles, cooked
½ cup	Garbanzo Beans/Chickpeas, boiled
1 tablespoon	Feta Cheese
¼ cup	Sweet Raw Green Bell Peppers, chopped
¼ cup	Deluxe Artichoke Hearts
¼ cup	Tomato, chopped
¼ cup	Raw Celery, chopped
¼ cup	Low-Calorie Salad Dressing, oil-free
1 tablespoon	Fresh Lemon Juice
½ each	Whole-Wheat Pita Pocket Bread

Calories	488
Nutrient Breakdown	
• Protein	20 grams
• Carbohydrates	89 grams
• Fat	8 grams
Saturated Fat	3 grams

Recipe Tip:
The sharp flavor of cheese is a great taste enhancer. Try using Parmesan, Romano, or Gorgonzola for an equally tantalizing flavor.

Spicy Oven-Fried Chicken

3 ounces	Spicy Oven-Fried Chicken (recipe p. 152)
10 ounces	Sweet Potato, peeled after baking
1 cup	Green Snap/String Beans, raw or boiled

Calories	525
Nutrient Breakdown	
• Protein	28 grams
• Carbohydrates	92 grams
• Fat	6 grams
Saturated Fat	1 gram

Recipe Tip:
Do you prefer dark meat? Try skinless drumsticks. They contain a mere 28% calories from fat while skinless thighs yield 47% calories from fat.

Pasta Primavera

1 cup	Rotini Pasta Noodles, cooked
¼ cup	Garbanzo Beans/Chickpeas, dry or boiled
¼ cup	Red Kidney Beans, dry or boiled
½ cup	Italian Green Beans, frozen or boiled
¼ cup	Zucchini Squash, boiled
¼ cup	Tomato, chopped
½ cup	Spaghetti with Marinara Sauce
1 tablespoon	Parmesan Cheese, grated

Calories	478
Nutrient Breakdown	
• Protein	21 grams
• Carbohydrates	82 grams
• Fat	9 grams
Saturated Fat	2 grams

Recipe Tip:
Enjoy any mix of vegetables. A variety of green, yellow, and red bell peppers is another great combination.

Dijon Parmesan Halibut

3 ounces	Dijon Parmesan Halibut (recipe p. 157)
1½ cups	Long-Grain Brown Rice, cooked, hot
1 cup	Broccoli Pieces, boiled

Calories	**471**	
Nutrient Breakdown		
• Protein	28 grams	
• Carbohydrates	77 grams	
• Fat	6 grams	
Saturated Fat	1 gram	

Recipe Tip:
Any firm-fleshed fish will do: try swordfish, sea bass, or orange roughy.

Broccoli Tofu Stir-Fry

| 6 ounces | Broccoli Tofu Stir-Fry (recipe p. 154) |
| 2 cups | Long-Grain Rice, cooked |

Calories	**511**	
Nutrient Breakdown		
• Protein	22 grams	
• Carbohydrates	86 grams	
• Fat	8 grams	
Saturated Fat	1 gram	

Recipe Tip:
Any lean protein can be substituted for the tofu: lean sirloin beef, trimmed pork tenderloin, skinless chicken, or turkey.

Poached Salmon with Mustard-Ginger Sauce

2 ounces	Poached Salmon with Mustard Ginger Sauce (recipe p. 151)
8 ounces	Roasted Potato
1 cup	Deluxe Sugar Snap Peas

Calories	**508**
Nutrient Breakdown	
• Protein	25 grams
• Carbohydrates	90 grams
• Fat	6 grams
Saturated Fat	1 gram

Recipe Tip:
For a great summer treat, try substituting corn on the cob for the roasted potatoes.

Flank Steak Dinner

2 ounces	Beef Flank Steak (choice), broiled
8 ounces	Garlicky Mashed Potatoes (recipe p. 148)
2 cups	Mixed Salad Greens/Lettuce
2 tablespoons	Fat-Free Italian Dressing
2 medium slices	French Bread

Calories	**504**
Nutrient Breakdown	
• Protein	26 grams
• Carbohydrates	80 grams
• Fat	9 grams
Saturated Fat	3 grams

Recipe Tip:
Flank is not the only lean meat great on the grill or broiled. Other options include: top sirloin, London broil, filet mignon, or beef tenderloin.

South-of-the-Border Chili

12 ounces	South-of-the-Border Vegetarian Chili (recipe p. 150)
2 tablespoons	Part-Skim, Low-Moisture Mozzarella Cheese, shredded
2 ounces	French Bread
2 cups	Mixed Salad Greens/Lettuce
1 tablespoon	Low-Calorie Dressing, oil-free

Calories	**474**
Nutrient Breakdown	
• Protein	26 grams
• Carbohydrates	83 grams
• Fat	7 grams
Saturated Fat	2 grams

Recipe Tip:
If you're not a beef lover, you can easily use ground turkey in this recipe.

Seafood Pizza

1 slice	Seafood Pizza (recipe p. 153)
2 cups	Tossed Green Salad
½ each	Medium Whole Tomato
5 slices	Cucumber with Peel
2 tablespoons	Fat-Free Italian Dressing
2 medium slices	French Bread

Calories	**487**
Nutrient Breakdown	
• Protein	20 grams
• Carbohydrates	85 grams
• Fat	8 grams
Saturated Fat	3 grams

Recipe Tip:
Are you a traditionalist? A great low-fat pizza topping is Canadian bacon. Made from pork tenderloin, it has the same fat content as skinless chicken breast.

Black Bean Soup

16 ounces	Black Bean Soup (recipe p. 155)
2 ounces	Mixed Grain Bread
2 cups	Mixed Salad Greens/Lettuce
1 tablespoon	Low-Calorie Italian Dressing
1 cup	Cantaloupe/Muskmelon, cubed
1 ounce	Part-Skim, Low-Moisture Mozzarella Cheese, shredded

Calories	**475**
Nutrient Breakdown	
• Protein	24 grams
• Carbohydrates	89 grams
• Fat	5 grams
Saturated Fat	1 gram

Recipe Tip:
Any bean, lentil, or split pea soup will work in this meal plan.

Meal Plan #3–THE HUNTER-GATHERER

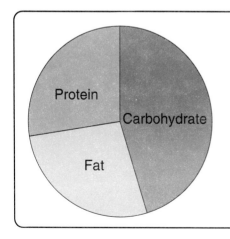

Meal Plan #3—
THE HUNTER-GATHERER

Carbohydrate	45 to 50%
Fat	25 to 30%
Protein	25 to 30%

Breakfast Options

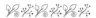

Oatmeal Blueberry Pancake Breakfast

2 each	Oatmeal Blueberry Pancakes (recipe p. 143) with 2 tablespoons Maple Syrup
4 ounces	Whole Ham, roasted, trimmed
¾ cup	Fresh Berries
2 tablespoons	Dried English Walnuts, chopped

Calories	534
Nutrient Breakdown	
• Protein	36 grams
• Carbohydrates	63 grams
• Fat	17 grams
Saturated Fat	3 grams

Recipe Tip:
You can easily substitute any berry, apples, or bananas in the pancake recipe. Also, you may substitute Canadian bacon, a lean hamburger patty, or minute steak.

Breakfast Quesadilla and Melon

3 each	Corn Tortillas
¾ ounce	Part-Skim, Low-Moisture Mozzarella Cheese, shredded
2 ounce-weight	Skinless Chicken Breast, roasted
2 tablespoons	Salsa
1 cup	Cantaloupe/Muskmelon, cubed

Calories	481
Nutrient Breakdown	
• Protein	34 grams
• Carbohydrates	59 grams
• Fat	14 grams
Saturated Fat	6 grams

Recipe Tip:
If you prefer flour tortillas substitute 1 10-inch flour tortilla for every 2 corn tortillas.

Apple Brunch Breakfast

4 ounces	Apple Brunch Corn Cakes (recipe p. 144)
8 ounces	2% Low-Fat Cottage Cheese
½ cup	Fresh Fruit Salad
1 teaspoon	Butter

Calories	485
Nutrient Breakdown	
• Protein	36 grams
• Carbohydrates	56 grams
• Fat	14 grams
Saturated Fat	6 grams

Recipe Tip:
Anytime fresh fruit salad is included in a menu plan you can substitute 1 cup of any cut-up fresh fruit.

Cold Cereal Breakfast

1 cup	Shredded Wheat Cereal, small biscuit
1 cup	2% Lower-Fat Milk
1 cup	Whole Strawberries
4 tablespoons	Dried Black Walnuts

Calories	507
Nutrient Breakdown	
• Protein	21 grams
• Carbohydrates	60 grams
• Fat	24 grams
Saturated Fat	4 grams

Recipe Tip:
Substitute any cold cereal:
• 2 cups shredded wheat is equivalent to 3 ounces of other cold cereals.
• 1 ½ cups shredded wheat is equivalent to 2 ¼ ounces other cold cereals.

Bagel and Lox Breakfast

3 ounces   Plain Bagel
4 tablespoons Low-Fat Cream Cheese
4 ounces   Smoked Chinook Salmon/Lox
½ cup   Fresh Fruit Salad

Calories	**518**
Nutrient Breakdown	
• Protein	32 grams
• Carbohydrates	59 grams
• Fat	17 grams
Saturated Fat	7 grams

Recipe Tip:
Instead of salmon lox enjoy other smoked fish or lean deli meats. They work just as well and offer more variety.

Peanut Butter Toast Breakfast

2 slices   Cracked Wheat Bread
2½ tablespoons Chunky Peanut Butter
1¼ cups   Fresh Fruit Salad

Calories	**491**
Nutrient Breakdown	
• Protein	15 grams
• Carbohydrates	66 grams
• Fat	23 grams
Saturated Fat	4 grams

Recipe Tip:
Using peanut butter in a meal means your fat content will be higher than usual. Because the fats in nuts and seeds are primarily unsaturated, any nut butter will work here. Enjoy the convenience!

Oatmeal Breakfast

1½ cups	Oatmeal Cereal, cooked
1 cup	Low-Fat Yogurt, plain
2 tablespoons	Dried Black Walnuts
1 tablespoon	Seedless Raisins, packed

Calories	498
Nutrient Breakdown	
• Protein	26 grams
• Carbohydrates	65 grams
• Fat	16 grams
Saturated Fat	4 grams

Recipe Tip:
Use any favorite dried fruit in your oatmeal. For a heartier consistency try using steel-cut oats.

Eggs and Toast

3 each	Eggs, cooked without fat
2 slices	Cracked Wheat Bread
1 cup	Fresh Fruit Salad
½ tablespoon	Jam

Calories	488
Nutrient Breakdown	
• Protein	24 grams
• Carbohydrates	59 grams
• Fat	19 grams
Saturated Fat	5 grams

Recipe Tip:
Any type of bread can be used in this meal (i.e., sourdough, whole grain, rye, oatmeal, pumpernickel). English muffins work well, too.

❦ ❦ ❦ ❦

Waffles and Fruit

2 each   Waffles, frozen or toasted
½ cup   Fresh Strawberries, sliced
4 ounces   Whole Ham, roasted, trimmed
2 tablespoons   Maple Syrup

Calories	493
Nutrient Breakdown	
• Protein	33 grams
• Carbohydrates	61 grams
• Fat	12 grams
Saturated Fat	3 grams

Recipe Tip:
Waffles made at home or ordered from a restaurant are larger than typical frozen waffles. You'll probably need to moderate your portion.

❦ ❦ ❦ ❦

French Toast

2 slices   Cracked Wheat Bread
2 each   Raw Egg Whites
½ teaspoon   Corn Oil (for cooking)
2 ounces   Ham Dinner Steak, water added
1 cup   Fresh Fruit Salad
½ tablespoon   Maple Syrup

Calories	509
Nutrient Breakdown	
• Protein	30 grams
• Carbohydrates	59 grams
• Fat	18 grams
Saturated Fat	5 grams

Recipe Tip:
Enhance with a variety of bread. One day use whole wheat, other days sourdough or French. For special occasions, cinnamon-raisin bread.

Lunch and Dinner Options

BBQ Chicken on a Bun

1 each	Mixed Grain Hamburger/Hot Dog Bun
3 ounces	Skinless Chicken Breast, roasted
2 tablespoons	Barbecue Sauce
5 each	Baby Carrots, raw 2.75 inch
1 cup	Fresh Fruit Salad
1 tablespoon	Ranch Salad Dressing

Calories	451
Nutrient Breakdown	
• Protein	33 grams
• Carbohydrates	54 grams
• Fat	13 grams
Saturated Fat	3 grams

Recipe Tip:
Lean roast beef and pork tenderloin also work well in this sandwich. Be sure to not overcook the pork. The pork is done when juices run clear.

Oriental Turkey Express

5 ounces	Turkey Breast, cooked
2 teaspoons	Sesame Oil (drizzle over stir-fry vegetables for extra flavor)
¼ cup	Szechwan Sauce
1 cup	Japanese Stir-Fry Vegetables
¾ cup	Long-Grain Rice, cooked

Calories	518
Nutrient Breakdown	
• Protein	37 grams
• Carbohydrates	66 grams
• Fat	13 grams
Saturated Fat	2 grams

Recipe Tip:
You can use a variety of Asian seasonings to enhance this dish. Hoisan sauce will give it a sweeter flavor while a black bean sauce is a very savory option.

Soup and Sandwich

8 ounces	Lentil Soup
2 slices	Cracked Wheat Bread
3 ounces	Beef Round-Eye (choice)—Lean Roast Beef, trimmed
1 each	Medium Orange
½ tablespoon	Mayonnaise

Calories	510
Nutrient Breakdown	
• Protein	37 grams
• Carbohydrates	60 grams
• Fat	14 grams
Saturated Fat	3 grams

Recipe Tip:

This combination has endless possibilities. Any hearty soup will complement the sandwich nicely. This sandwich can be equally versatile. Try using sliced ham, turkey, or tuna salad.

Tuna Tostada Meal

1 each	Light and Healthy Tuna Tostada (recipe p. 149)
8 each	Baked Tortilla Chips
1 cup	Fresh Fruit Salad
2 tablespoons	Dried English Walnuts

Calories	529
Nutrient Breakdown	
• Protein	33 grams
• Carbohydrates	66 grams
• Fat	17 grams
Saturated Fat	2 grams

Recipe Tip:

For an exotic touch, try using crab, shrimp, squid, or lobster. These are equally low-fat protein sources.

Grilled Hamburger

4 ounces	Beef Round-Eye (choice)
1 each	Hamburger Bun
2 leaves	Iceberg/Crisphead Lettuce
2 slices	Fresh Tomato
1 slice	Red Onion
1 tablespoon	Prepared Mustard
1 tablespoon	Low-Calorie Mayonnaise
5 slices	Dill Pickle
1 cup	Fresh Fruit Salad

Calories	501
Nutrient Breakdown	
• Protein	40 grams
• Carbohydrates	57 grams
• Fat	13 grams
Saturated Fat	4 grams

Recipe Tip:
The leanest ground beef (7% fat by weight) may not hold together well, so try adding an egg white to the raw meat before shaping it into patties.

Steak Lovers' Salad

3 ounces	Beef Tenderloin Steak, broiled
4 cups	Mixed Salad Greens/Lettuce
1 ounce	Honey Dijon Dressing (recipe p. 158)
2 ounces	Sourdough Roll
2 cups	Whole Strawberries

Calories	506
Nutrient Breakdown	
• Protein	35 grams
• Carbohydrates	62 grams
• Fat	15 grams
Saturated Fat	4 grams

Recipe Tip:
This is a great way to enjoy leftover grilled steak. Of course, grilled chicken or pork can work equally well.

Curried Chicken-Cilantro Salad

7½ ounces	Curried Chicken-Cilantro Salad (recipe p. 146)
2 ounces	Hard White Roll
1 cup	Fresh Fruit Salad

Calories 517
Nutrient Breakdown
• Protein 30 grams
• Carbohydrates 67 grams
• Fat 16 grams
Saturated Fat 3 grams

Recipe Tip:
For an easy on-the-go meal try stuffing the chicken-cilantro salad into a pita or rolling it into a tortilla or a piece of lavosh bread.

Speedy Salad Burritos

½ cup	Refried Beans, canned
2 each	Whole-Wheat Tortillas
2 ounces	Skinless Chicken Breast, roasted
¼ cup	Cheddar Cheese, shredded
1 cup	Iceberg/Crisphead Lettuce, chopped
¼ cup	Salsa

Calories 517
Nutrient Breakdown
• Protein 39 grams
• Carbohydrates 69 grams
• Fat 14 grams
Saturated Fat 7 grams

Recipe Tip:
Refried beans aren't the high-fat product most assume. One national brand is only 9% calories from fat. Refried black beans can also be used.

❧❧❧❧❧❧

Zesty Low-Fat Spinach Salad

1 each	Zesty Spinach Salad (recipe p. 147)
4 ounces	Honey Roast Turkey Breast

Calories	489
Nutrient Breakdown	
• Protein	29 grams
• Carbohydrates	64 grams
• Fat	17 grams
Saturated Fat	3 grams

Recipe Tip:
Other grain options include bulgur, couscous, or a mix of brown and wild rice. Remember, brown rice takes a bit longer to cook than other grains.

❧❧❧❧❧❧

Veggie Pita Pizza

1½ each	Whole-Wheat Pita Pocket Bread
¼ cup	Tomato Sauce, canned
¼ cup	Sweet Green Bell Peppers, raw, chopped
¼ cup	Onions, raw, chopped
¼ cup	Mushroom Pieces, raw
¾ cup	Part-Skim, Low-Moisture Mozzarella Cheese, shredded
2 ounces	Canadian Bacon, unheated
2 cups	Tossed Green Salad
5 slices	Cucumber with Peel
¼ cup	Tomato, chopped
1 tablespoon	Low-Calorie Dressing, oil-free

Calories	495
Nutrient Breakdown	
• Protein	34 grams
• Carbohydrates	62 grams
• Fat	15 grams
Saturated Fat	6 grams

Recipe Tip:
Many other breads work well in this recipe. Boboli, sliced French bread, and sourdough rolls are good options.

Mediterranean Pasta Salad

1 cup	Rotini Pasta Noodles, cooked
¼ cup	Garbanzo Beans/Chickpeas, boiled
1 tablespoon	Feta Cheese
4 ounces	Squid (Philippine), boiled
¼ cup	Sweet Raw Green Bell Peppers, chopped
¼ cup	Deluxe Artichoke Hearts
¼ cup	Tomato, chopped
¼ cup	Raw Celery, chopped
¼ cup	Low-Calorie Salad Dressing, oil-free
1 tablespoon	Fresh Lemon Juice

Calories	505
Nutrient Breakdown	
• Protein	34 grams
• Carbohydrates	64 grams
• Fat	13 grams
Saturated Fat	3 grams

Recipe Tip:
The sharp flavor of cheese is a great taste enhancer. Try using Parmesan, Romano, or Gorgonzola for an equally tantalizing flavor.

Black Bean Soup

12 ounces	Black Bean Soup (recipe p. 155)
3 tablespoons	Asiago or Parmesan Cheese, shredded
1 ounce	Mixed Grain Bread
1 ounce	Part-Skim, Low-Moisture Mozzarella Cheese, shredded (Add cheese to salad for extra flavor or simply melt on bread for a cheesy treat.)
2 cups	Mixed Salad Greens/Lettuce
1 tablespoon	Low-Calorie Italian Dressing
1 cup	Cantaloupe/Muskmelon, cubed

Calories	499
Nutrient Breakdown	
• Protein	31 grams
• Carbohydrates	66 grams
• Fat	15 grams
Saturated Fat	7 grams

Recipe Tip:
Any bean, lentil, or split pea soup will work in this meal plan.

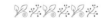

South-of-the-Border Chili

8 ounces	South-of-the-Border Vegetarian Chili (recipe p. 150)
2 ounces	Beef Roast, braised, trimmed
3 tablespoons	Cheddar Cheese, shredded
1½ medium slices	French Bread
2 cups	Mixed Salad Greens/Lettuce
1 tablespoon	Low-Calorie Dressing, oil-free

Calories	506
Nutrient Breakdown	
• Protein	39 grams
• Carbohydrates	59 grams
• Fat	14 grams
Saturated Fat	6 grams

Recipe Tip:
If you're not a beef lover, you can easily use ground turkey in this recipe.

Seafood Pizza Dinner

2 slices	Seafood Pizza (recipe p. 153)
2 cups	Tossed Green Salad
½ each	Medium Whole Tomato
5 slices	Cucumber with Peel
1 tablespoon	Italian Dressing
4 each	Shrimp, medium size, baked or broiled (Add additional shrimp to salad or pizza.)

Calories	564
Nutrient Breakdown	
• Protein	29 grams
• Carbohydrates	72 grams
• Fat	19 grams
Saturated Fat	5 grams

Recipe Tip:
Are you a traditionalist? A great low-fat pizza topping is Canadian bacon. Made from pork tenderloin, it has the same fat content as skinless chicken breast.

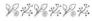

Poached Salmon with Mustard-Ginger Sauce

4 ounces	Poached Salmon with Mustard-Ginger Sauce (recipe p. 151)
4 ounces	Roasted Potato
1 teaspoon	Olive Oil (Drizzle over potato or snap peas for extra flavor.)
1 cup	Deluxe Sugar Snap Peas

Calories	493
Nutrient Breakdown	
• Protein	33 grams
• Carbohydrates	56 grams
• Fat	15 grams
Saturated Fat	2 grams

Recipe Tip:
For a great summer treat, try substituting corn on the cob for the roasted potatoes.

Flank Steak Dinner

4 ounces	Beef Flank Steak (choice), broiled
6 ounces	Garlicky Mashed Potatoes (recipe p. 148)
2 cups	Mixed Salad Greens/Lettuce
2 tablespoons	Fat-Free Italian Dressing
1 medium slice	French Bread

Calories	498
Nutrient Breakdown	
• Protein	38 grams
• Carbohydrates	55 grams
• Fat	13 grams
Saturated Fat	5 grams

Recipe Tip:
Flank is not the only lean meat great on the grill or broiled. Other options include: top sirloin, London broil, filet mignon, or beef tenderloin.

Dijon Parmesan Halibut

4 ounces	Dijon Parmesan Halibut (recipe p. 157)
1 cup	Long-Grain Brown Rice, cooked, hot
1 cup	Broccoli Pieces, boiled
2 cups	Mixed Green Salad/Lettuce
1 tablespoon	Low-Calorie Italian Dressing

Calories	486
Nutrient Breakdown	
• Protein	32 grams
• Carbohydrates	60 grams
• Fat	14 grams
Saturated Fat	2 grams

Recipe Tip:
Any firm-fleshed fish will do: try swordfish, sea bass, or orange roughy.

Broccoli Tofu Stir-Fry

10 ounces	Broccoli Tofu Stir-Fry (recipe p. 154)
1¼ cups	Long-Grain Rice, cooked

Calories	493
Nutrient Breakdown	
• Protein	25 grams
• Carbohydrates	63 grams
• Fat	18 grams
Saturated Fat	3 grams

Recipe Tip:
Any lean protein can be substituted for the tofu: lean sirloin beef, trimmed pork tenderloin, skinless chicken, or turkey.

Spicy Oven-Fried Chicken

5 ounces	Spicy Oven-Fried Chicken (recipe p. 152)
4 ounces	Sweet Potato, peeled after baking
1 cup	Green Snap/String Beans, raw, boiled
1 teaspoon	Butter

Calories	510
Nutrient Breakdown	
• Protein	39 grams
• Carbohydrates	59 grams
• Fat	13 grams
Saturated Fat	4 grams

Recipe Tip:
Do you prefer dark meat? Try skinless drumsticks. They contain a mere 28% calories from fat while skinless thighs yield 47% calories from fat.

Pasta Primavera

1 cup	Rotini Pasta Noodles, cooked
1 tablespoon	Garbanzo Beans/Chickpeas, dry, boiled
1 tablespoon	Red Kidney Beans, dry, boiled
½ cup	Italian Green Beans, frozen, boiled
¼ cup	Zucchini Squash, boiled

¼ cup	Tomato, chopped
½ cup	Spaghetti with Marinara Sauce
2 tablespoons	Parmesan Cheese, grated
2 ounces	Skinless Chicken Meat, roasted

Calories   521
Nutrient Breakdown
• Protein   34 grams
• Carbohydrates   67 grams
• Fat   14 grams
  Saturated Fat   4 grams

Recipe Tip:
Enjoy any mix of vegetables. A variety of green, yellow, and red bell peppers is another great combination.

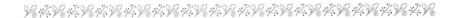

RECIPES

Oatmeal Blueberry Pancakes

¾   *cup steel-cut oats*
¾   *cup whole-wheat pastry flour*
2   *teaspoons aluminum-free baking powder*
½   *teaspoon baking soda*
½   *teaspoon salt (optional)*
1½   *cups buttermilk*
1   *large egg, lightly beaten*
2   *tablespoons, plus approximately 1 tablespoon, vegetable oil (such as canola, safflower, or sunflower)*
½   *cup blueberries*

1. In a large bowl, combine the oats, flour, baking powder, baking soda, and salt, if using.

2. In a small bowl, stir together the buttermilk, egg, and oil.

3. Fold the liquid ingredients into the dry, and mix until smooth. You can add more liquid for thinner pancakes. Gently fold in blueberries.

4. Over medium-high heat, brush a skillet or griddle with vegetable oil, and when the oil is hot, drop ¼ cup of the batter onto the skillet. Using a spatula, spread out the batter to the desired thickness.

5. Add as many pancakes to the skillet as will easily fit. Cook the pancakes until they are bubbly on top and brown on the bottom, about 3 minutes. Then flip them and cook briefly on the other side, about 2 minutes. Add a bit more oil to the skillet as needed. Repeat with the remaining batter.

Makes 18 pancakes.

PREPARATION TIME: 10 minutes

COOKING TIME: 15 to 20 minutes

Serving size: 1 pancake (approx. 1½ ounces)		Fat—Total:	3 g
Calories:	71	Saturated:	½ g
Protein:	3 g	Unsaturated:	2 g
Carbohydrates:	10 g	Dietary Fiber:	1 g

Apple Brunch Corn Cakes

APPLE TOPPING

1   *tablespoon vegetable oil (such as canola, safflower, or sunflower)*

2   *tablespoons pure maple syrup*

½   *teaspoon ground cinnamon*

2   *large Golden or Red Delicious apples, peeled, cored, and sliced ¼-inch thick (3 cups)*

CORN BREAD

¾   cup ground yellow or blue cornmeal
¾   cup whole-wheat pastry flour
1   teaspoon aluminum-free baking powder
½   teaspoon salt (optional)
¼   teaspoon baking soda
1   large egg, lightly beaten
1   cup buttermilk, or ½ cup nonfat plain yogurt plus ½ cup
     skim or soy milk
¼   cup pure maple syrup
1   tablespoon vegetable oil (such as canola, safflower, or
     sunflower)

1. Preheat the oven to 375° F.

2. In a 10-inch, heavy ovenproof skillet (cast iron is preferable), combine the oil, maple syrup, and cinnamon, and stir over medium-high heat until hot.

3. Add the apple slices and sauté, tossing occasionally, until slightly softened, 5 to 7 minutes.

4. Remove the skillet from the heat. Arrange the apple slices in an attractive pattern in the skillet, fanning them out from the center. Set aside.

5. In a large bowl, combine the cornmeal, flour, baking powder, salt, if using, and baking soda.

6. In a small bowl, whisk together the egg, buttermilk, or yogurt/milk mixture, syrup, and oil.

7. Make a well in the center of the dry ingredients, pour in the liquid mixture, and stir together just until combined, being careful not to overmix.

8. Spread the batter gently over the apples and bake the corn bread for 30 to 35 minutes, or until a wooden toothpick inserted in the center comes out clean.

9. Cool the corn bread in the skillet on a wire rack for about 5 minutes, then invert onto a serving plate, rearranging any apple slices that stick to the pan. Serve immediately.

MAKES 8 SERVINGS.

PREPARATION TIME: 20 minutes
BAKING TIME: 30 to 35 minutes

Serving size: 1 4-ounce piece		Fat—Total:	5 g
Calories:	197	Saturated:	1 g
Protein:	5 g	Unsaturated:	4 g
Carbohydrates:	35 g	Dietary Fiber:	3 g

Curried Chicken-Cilantro Salad

LEMON CURRY DRESSING

2   *tablespoons extra-virgin olive oil*
3   *tablespoons fresh lemon juice*
3   *tablespoons reduced-fat mayonnaise*
2   *teaspoons honey*
2   *teaspoons curry powder*
2   *tablespoons chopped fresh basil, or 1 to 2 teaspoons dried*
¼   *teaspoon sea salt (optional)*

2   *cups cooked skinless chicken, cut into bite-size pieces*
2   *cups romaine or green leaf lettuce, washed, dried, and torn into bite-size pieces*
2   *cups red leaf lettuce, washed, dried, and torn into bite-size pieces*
1   *cup baby field greens, or any other greens desired, washed and dried*
1   *cup chopped fresh cilantro*
½   *cup chopped red onion*
½   *cup chopped green onion*

1. In a small bowl, whisk together the dressing ingredients. Add the chicken to the dressing and toss to coat. Chill until ready to serve.

2. In a large bowl, combine the lettuces and greens, cilantro, and red and green onions. Just before serving, add the chicken and dressing, toss to mix, and serve immediately.

Makes 4 servings.

PREPARATION TIME: 20 minutes

Serving size: 6 ounces		Fat—Total:	10 g
Calories:	201	Saturated:	2 g
Protein:	19 g	Unsaturated:	8 g
Carbohydrates:	9 g	Dietary Fiber:	2 g

Zesty Spinach Salad

1   cup cooked brown rice
2   medium carrots, scrubbed and grated

DRESSING

Juice and zest of 1½ lemons
1   tablespoon extra-virgin olive oil
2   tablespoons finely chopped fresh basil, or 2 teaspoons
        dried
1   large garlic clove, pressed
1   teaspoon honey
    Pinch of cayenne pepper
    Pinch of sea salt (optional)

1   bunch fresh spinach, washed, drained, and torn into
        bite-size pieces

1. In a large salad bowl, combine the brown rice and carrots.

2. In a small bowl, whisk together the lemon juice and zest, olive oil, basil, garlic, honey, cayenne, and sea salt, if using. Pour the dressing over the rice mixture and combine well.

3. Just before serving, toss in the spinach, mixing gently.

Mᴀᴋᴇs 1 sᴇʀᴠɪɴɢ.

PREPARATION TIME: 15 minutes

Serving size: 13 ounces		Fat—Total:	15 g
Calories:	376	Saturated:	2 g
Protein:	8 g	Unsaturated:	13 g
Carbohydrates:	59 g	Dietary Fiber:	7 g

Garlicky Mashed Potatoes

2   *large heads garlic*
     Extra-virgin olive oil, for drizzling
½   *cup vegetable stock or water*
3   *pounds russet potatoes, peeled and quartered*
½   *cup skim milk*
     Salt and freshly ground black pepper to taste (optional)

1. Preheat the oven to 350° F.

2. Remove the outer papery skin from the heads of the garlic, then place the garlic in a small baking pan and drizzle with a bit of olive oil. Pour the stock into the pan. Cover with foil or a lid, and bake until the garlic is very soft when squeezed, about 1 hour. Remove from the oven, and let it cool slightly. The soft garlic will come out of the skins very easily.

3. While the garlic is baking, place the potatoes in a 5- or 6-quart pan with enough water to cover them by 1 inch. Cover the pan and bring the water to a boil over high heat. Reduce the heat and continue boiling gently until the potatoes are tender when pierced with a fork, about 20 minutes. Drain well.

4. When cool enough to handle, cut the garlic heads in half crosswise and squeeze the soft garlic interiors into a large bowl. Beat the garlic with an electric mixer until smooth.

5. Add the hot potatoes and milk, and beat again until smooth; add salt and pepper, if using. Serve immediately.

Makes 6 servings.

PREPARATION TIME: 15 minutes

COOKING TIME: 1 hour

Serving size: 8 ounces		Fat—Total:	1 g
Calories:	182	Saturated:	<1 g
Protein:	4 g	Unsaturated:	<1 g
Carbohydrates:	40 g	Dietary Fiber:	3 g

Light and Healthy Tuna Tostada

1   *12½-ounce can water-packed tuna, drained*
½   *cup finely chopped onion*
1   *large tomato, chopped in medium chunks*
    Sea salt and freshly ground pepper to taste (optional)
3   *tablespoons plain nonfat yogurt*
2–3 *tablespoons fresh lime juice*
2   *teaspoons hot sauce*
4   *corn tortillas (flour can be substituted, but it's not as good)*
1   *teaspoon extra-virgin olive oil*
¾   *cup vegetarian refried beans (optional)*
2   *cups chopped mixed salad greens*
¾   *cup chopped fresh cilantro*

1. In a medium bowl, combine the tuna, small onion, and tomato; add salt and pepper, if using. In a small bowl, whisk together the yogurt, lime juice, and hot sauce; add to the tuna and mix well. Cover and chill if not serving immediately.

2. Preheat the oven to 375° F.

3. Lightly oil a cookie sheet, arrange the tortillas on the sheet, and brush the tops lightly with oil. Bake just until golden, about 10 minutes. Remove from oven, and arrange tortillas on individual plates.

4. Spread the tortillas with a layer of refried beans, if using. Sprinkle the mixed salad greens over the beans. Add a layer of the tuna mixture, and top with the cilantro.

Makes 4 servings.

PREPARATION TIME: 20 to 25 minutes

Serving size: 1 10-ounce tostada		Fat—Total:	3 g
Calories:	259	Saturated:	1 g
Protein:	29 g	Unsaturated:	2 g
Carbohydrates:	29 g	Dietary Fiber:	5 g

South-of-the-Border Vegetarian Chili

1   16-ounce can red kidney beans, drained
1   16-ounce can pinto beans, drained
2–3 cups vegetable stock or water
2   14-ounce cans whole tomatoes
2   cups chopped onion
1   cup frozen corn
1½   cups chopped green bell pepper
4   garlic cloves, minced
3   tablespoons chili powder
1   tablespoon ground cumin
1   teaspoon dried oregano
1   small green chile, diced (remove the seeds)
2   teaspoons salt (optional)

1. In a large soup pot or Dutch oven, cover the beans with stock or water and bring to a boil. Add the tomatoes, 1 cup onion, corn,

¾ cup green pepper, garlic, 2 tablespoons chili powder, cumin, and oregano. Reduce the heat and simmer for 1 hour and 30 minutes.

2. When the beans are tender, mash some of them with a wooden spoon or a potato masher. Add the remaining 1 cup onion, the remaining ¾ cup green pepper, and the green chile, and stir.

3. Cook for an additional 30 minutes. Add the remaining 1 tablespoon chili powder and the salt, if using, for the last 5 minutes of cooking.

Makes 8 servings.

PREPARATION TIME: 20 minutes
COOKING TIME: Approximately 2 hours

Serving size: 12 ounces		Fat—Total:	2 g
Calories:	256	Saturated:	<1 g
Protein:	15 g	Unsaturated:	1 g
Carbohydrates:	49 g	Dietary Fiber:	16 g

Poached Salmon with Mustard-Ginger Sauce

MUSTARD SAUCE

4   *tablespoons plain nonfat yogurt*
3   *teaspoons Dijon mustard*
1½   *teaspoons minced fresh ginger*
1   *teaspoon honey*
1   *pound salmon fillet, cut into 4 pieces, rinsed and*
        patted dry
      Minced fresh chives or parsley, for garnish

1. In a small bowl, combine the yogurt, mustard, ginger, and honey. Set aside while the fish cooks.

2. Cover the bottom of a large pan with about 2 inches of water. Bring the water to a gentle boil, and add the salmon. Reduce the

heat and simmer until the fish is opaque in the center, 8 to 10 minutes. Remove the fish from the pan, drain, and gently pat dry.

3. Arrange the salmon on a serving plate, and spoon the mustard sauce over the fish. Garnish with chives or parsley.

MAKES 4 SERVINGS.

PREPARATION TIME: 25 minutes
COOKING TIME: 10 minutes

Serving size: 3 ounces		Fat—Total:	8 g
Calories:	159	Saturated:	1 g
Protein:	19 g	Unsaturated:	7 g
Carbohydrates:	3 g	Dietary Fiber:	1 g

Spicy Oven-Fried Chicken

3   *tablespoons hot pepper sauce*
1   *tablespoon Worcestershire sauce*
1   *teaspoon salt (optional)*
1   *teaspoon freshly ground black pepper*
8   *chicken pieces (cut whole chicken or breast or thighs),*
     skinned, washed, and patted dry
2   *cups unseasoned bread crumbs*
1–2 *tablespoons vegetable oil (such as canola, safflower, or*
     sunflower)

1. In a large bowl, whisk together the hot sauce, Worcestershire sauce, salt, if using, and pepper. Add the chicken and marinate, covered, in the refrigerator from 2 to 24 hours.

2. Preheat the oven to 425° F.

3. Remove the chicken from the marinade and add the bread crumbs to the marinade. Mix well and coat the chicken thoroughly.

4. Spread the oil over the bottom of a shallow 9- x 13-inch baking dish. Arrange the chicken in the dish and bake for 15 to 20 minutes. Turn the chicken over, reduce the heat to 325° F, and

cook for an additional 15 to 20 minutes, or until the juices run clear when pierced with a fork.

MAKES 8 SERVINGS.

PREPARATION TIME: 10 minutes, plus time to marinate
BAKING TIME: 30 to 45 minutes

Serving size: 4 ounces		Fat—Total:	8 g
Calories:	274	Saturated:	2 g
Protein:	30 g	Unsaturated:	6 g
Carbohydrates:	19 g	Dietary Fiber:	1 g

Seafood Pizza

20   medium shrimp, peeled and deveined
      Premade dough or 1 large or 2 small Boboli pizza crust
½   cup tomato sauce
2   garlic cloves, minced
½–¾ cup grated part-skim mozzarella cheese
      Pinch of red pepper flakes
¼   cup chopped fresh cilantro leaves

1. Preheat the oven to 475° F.

2. In a small pot, braise the shrimp until they just barely turn pink or opaque, 3 to 4 minutes, and then set them aside.

3. On a well-floured surface, press out the pizza dough to form 1 12-inch or 2 6-inch pizza rounds. Lightly oil a black steel pan or cookie sheet, or use a baking stone sprinkled with cornmeal. Transfer the dough to the pizza pan.

4. Spread the tomato sauce over the dough, leaving a ½-inch rim.

5. Sprinkle the garlic over the sauce and top with the cheese.

6. Arrange the shrimp over the cheese.

7. Sprinkle a few red pepper flakes and cilantro on the top.

8. Place the pizza pan as close to the oven floor as possible and bake until the crust is golden brown, about 15 minutes.

Makes 4 servings.

PREPARATION TIME: 10 to 15 minutes
BAKING TIME: 15 minutes

Serving size: 1 3-ounce piece		Fat—Total:	5 g
Calories:	200	Saturated:	2 g
Protein:	10 g	Unsaturated:	3 g
Carbohydrates:	28 g	Dietary Fiber:	1 g

Broccoli Tofu Stir-Fry

1   pound firm tofu
1   tablespoon extra-virgin olive oil or toasted sesame oil
4   tablespoons minced fresh ginger
4   large garlic cloves, minced
½   medium white onion, sliced lengthwise into crescents
2   carrots, cut diagonally into ½-inch pieces
1   cup sliced mushrooms
1½ cups broccoli florets
2   cups chopped Chinese greens, such as bok choy or napa
    cabbage
½   small red bell pepper and ½ small yellow bell pepper, cut
    diagonally into strips
½   cup chopped red cabbage

SAUCE

¼   cup tamari or light soy sauce
3   tablespoons sesame seeds
2   tablespoons brown rice vinegar
1   tablespoon honey
1   tablespoon toasted sesame oil

1. Cut tofu into bite-size pieces.

2. Heat the oil in large skillet or wok over medium-high heat. Add the ginger and garlic and cook for 2 to 3 minutes. Add the onion, carrots, and tofu and cook for 2 minutes. Reduce the heat to medium, add the mushrooms, and cook for 3 additional minutes, or until the onion is transparent. Add the broccoli and cook 2 to 3 minutes, then add the greens, bell pepper, and red cabbage, and cook 2 minutes more.

3. To make the sauce, in a small bowl, combine the tamari, 2 tablespoons sesame seeds, rice vinegar, honey, and sesame oil. Add the sauce to the vegetable mixture in the skillet, and cook for 4 to 5 minutes over low heat.

4. Sprinkle the dish with the remaining tablespoon of sesame seeds, and serve hot with brown rice.

MAKES 4 SERVINGS.

PREPARATION TIME: 25 minutes

COOKING TIME: 20 minutes

Serving size: 10 ounces		Fat—Total:	18 g
Calories:	290	Saturated:	3 g
Protein:	20 g	Unsaturated:	15 g
Carbohydrates:	20 g	Dietary Fiber:	4 g

Black Bean Soup

2   cups black beans, soaked overnight and drained, or
     4 15-ounce cans black beans
6   cups water
1   large onion, chopped
3   garlic cloves, minced
1   cup fresh corn kernels, cut off the cob, or frozen corn
     (optional)
1   4 ½-ounce can diced green chilies, or 2 tablespoons diced
     fresh mild green chilies

¼   cup chopped fresh cilantro
2   tablespoons tomato paste
1   teaspoon ground cumin
1   teaspoon dried oregano
½   teaspoon chili powder
    Pinch of freshly ground black pepper
1   teaspoon salt (optional)

GARNISH OPTIONS

Chopped fresh cilantro
Minced onion
Crumbled baked tortilla chips

1. In a large soup pot or Dutch oven, combine the beans with the water, onion, and garlic, and bring to a boil. Reduce the heat and simmer, covered, for 1½ hours or until the beans are tender.

2. Stir in the corn, if using, chilies, cilantro, tomato paste, cumin, oregano, chili powder, and black pepper, and simmer, uncovered, for 30 minutes, or until the soup is somewhat thickened. The longer it is simmered, the thicker the soup will be. Add the salt, if using, at the very end.

3. Pour the soup into bowls, and top with any of the garnishes.

MAKES 4 TO 6 SERVINGS.

PREPARATION TIME: 20 to 25 minutes
COOKING TIME: 2 hours

Serving size: 16 ounces		Fat—Total:	1 g
Calories:	242	Saturated:	<1 g
Protein:	15 g	Unsaturated:	<1 g
Carbohydrates:	46 g	Dietary Fiber:	15 g

Dijon Parmesan Halibut

1–1½   pounds halibut, cut into 4 pieces
¼   cup fresh lemon juice
       Lemon pepper to taste
       Salt to taste (optional)

TOPPING

1   teaspoon reduced-fat mayonnaise
2   tablespoons finely grated low-fat Parmesan cheese
2   teaspoons fresh lemon juice
2   garlic cloves, pressed or finely minced
2   small green onions, thinly sliced
2   teaspoons Dijon mustard
¼   teaspoon hot sauce or pinch of cayenne pepper

1. On each side of each fish steak, make 3 diagonal cuts 2 inches long and ½-inch deep. Place the halibut in a large, shallow dish and pour the lemon juice over it. Marinate the halibut for 30 minutes at room temperature.

2. Preheat the oven to 450° F.

3. Place the fish on a broiling pan, and sprinkle with the marinade along with the lemon pepper. Bake the fish for 15 minutes, until it is opaque in the middle. Remove from the oven, and then turn the oven to broil.

4. While the halibut is baking, in a small bowl, combine the mayonnaise, Parmesan cheese, lemon juice, garlic, onion, mustard, and hot sauce or cayenne, and mix well.

5. If desired, sprinkle the fish with salt, then spread the topping over the fish. Broil the fish for about 1 minute, until the topping is golden brown.

Makes 4 servings.

PREPARATION TIME: 10 minutes, plus 30 minutes to marinate
COOKING TIME: 15 to 20 minutes

Serving size: 3 ounces		Fat—Total:	3 g
Calories:	104	Saturated:	1 g
Protein:	16 g	Unsaturated:	2 g
Carbohydrates:	2 g	Dietary Fiber:	<1 g

Steak Lovers' Salad

1   12-ounce steak (such as flank, chuck, or tenderloin)
1   large onion, sliced in rings

HONEY-DIJON DRESSING

2   tablespoons extra-virgin olive oil
4   tablespoons fresh lemon juice
2   teaspoons honey
1½ teaspoons Dijon mustard
½   teaspoon salt (optional)

½   head romaine lettuce, washed, dried, and torn into
      bite-size pieces
½   head red leaf lettuce, washed, dried, and torn into
      bite-size pieces

Note: Chicken or turkey can be substituted.

1. Preheat the grill or broiler.
2. Trim the fat from the steak, and grill or broil until medium to medium-well. Cool, cut into bite-size pieces, drain on a paper towel to absorb excess fat, and chill.
3. Grill or broil onion until tender, 6 to 8 minutes. Place onion slices on a paper towel and allow to cool.
4. In a small bowl, whisk together the olive oil, lemon juice, honey, mustard, and salt, if using.
5. In a large salad bowl, combine the steak, onion, and lettuces. Toss with the dressing, and serve immediately.

MAKES 4 SERVINGS.

PREPARATION TIME: 15 minutes
COOKING TIME: 15 to 20 minutes

		Fat—Total:	14 g
Serving size: 9 ounces		Saturated:	4 g
Calories:	280	Unsaturated:	10 g
Protein:	28 g	Dietary Fiber:	2 g
Carbohydrates:	10 g		

MOVING OUT OF YOUR "DIET" MENTALITY

I've noticed that most people tend to get caught in a vicious cycle of dieting and then blowing the diet. It usually begins something like this: You're unhappy with the way you look and feel. You seek a diet that promises instant weight loss through complete control of what, when, and how you eat. It feels safe, because you know exactly what you have to do to reach your goal. Soon enough you discover that you just can't stick to it . . . and you end up right back where you started, with the exact same eating pattern that got you wanting to go on a diet in the first place.

And so the cycle continues.

The problem here is that those "diets" treat the dieter like a machine that can be programmed. But the truth is that eating well has to take into account food's less scientific side.

You may yourself have already had an experience similar to this one. Maybe you, like millions of others, white-knuckled a liquid diet, or signed onto a program for which the food came preprepared. If you did, then it won't come as news to hear that the number-one reason people give up such diets is not because they reach their target weight. It's because they couldn't stand to go for so long without "real food." Anyway, it's simple human nature to rebel against such rigidity imposed from the outside. Being told what we're supposed to like, and to be satisfied with it, will eventually create its opposite intended effect.

I want to raise your awareness of those issues that get far too little attention when we preoccupy ourselves with grams of fat and calories—in fact, any single aspect of food.

Most plans don't take into account what food really means to us. They don't consider how the flavor and color and texture and temperature and presentation of food can give us so much pleasure. They don't consider how food is intimately entwined with our social and cultural customs. They don't consider how food and the environment in which we eat comfort us. They don't consider how eating foods that you don't like leaves you unsatisfied.

You need to recognize that eating well has to be seen as an ongoing process in your life. Ask yourself whether food contributes to your sense of well-being. Do you feel satisfied after eating? Do you feel nourished, able to physically meet the demands of your day? Do you like your food? Are you eating food that pleases you? The more frequently you can answer yes to any of those questions, the more functional your food is.

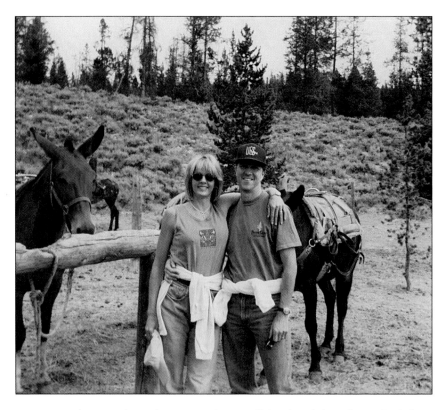

Steve and I on a three-day mountain expedition in Idaho. The mules help take up supplies. The rest is up to us.

Your ongoing process of learning to eat functionally enables you to explore your own needs and adjust your food choices accordingly. Here's what it means to enjoy independent eating, courtesy of my friend, nutritionist Bonnie Modugno, M.S., R.D.:

- Eating when you're hungry and stopping when you feel satisfied.
- Enjoying foods you truly love to eat.
- Choosing foods that enhance your physiological well-being.
- Knowing that the next time you get hungry, you have the opportunity to nourish and nurture yourself again.

Start by considering each meal a series of options. When you get good results from a meal—that is, when you feel satisfied and you know your nutritional needs have been met—you can make a note that that option was a keeper. And when a meal doesn't work, you make a note of that, too. While I love to experiment, I try always to avoid making mistakes I've made in the past, and I love repeating successes.

The process of making functional food choices begins with some honest self-assessment. You have to look carefully and precisely at where you are now, not where you want to be or think you should be. Start by examining the following scale of food behavior. It's arranged with least functional eating habits first, progressing up the scale, all the way to optimum eating.

Do you see yourself or your food behaviors described in any of these five prototypes?

Functional Food Systems: Five Levels to Optimal Eating

Level 5: Out-of-Control Eating

You feel completely out of control with food, and are probably in pain. You're either eating everything in sight, or you regularly binge and purge. You try to eat nothing at all, or you eat compulsively. Bottom line: What you eat and how you eat have little or nothing to do with your physiological/physical needs. You're so far from eating functionally that you probably can't remember a time when you did. And yet, you hang on to this food pattern because it's familiar to you—which is the only comfort you now get from food. The thought of changing is utterly terrifying.

Level 4: Rigidly Controlled Eating

Your entire food focus is viewed through the lens of being "on the program" or "off the program." In other words, you're either white-knuckling your way through a diet, or sliding out of control to Level 5. Not only that, but your pendulum swings even wider between being on and off a program. You can adhere to a diet for short periods, but find it impossible to live with. Still, you're convinced that if you could only find enough willpower or self-control to stay on a particular food plan—any plan!—success would be yours: you'd reach your target weight and stay there forever. Basically, you're drowning in a flood of wishful thinking; somewhere out there is the perfect diet for you—and someday you're going to find it.

LEVEL 3: EATING BY THE RULES

You know enough to know how you should be eating, and you've experienced from time to time how proper eating improves your whole outlook. Because of that, you're motivated to be "good," but you resent all those rules telling you what to eat and what not to eat. You believe you're doing the right thing, eating by the rules. But you're so busy being good, you don't give yourself permission to eat what you want. And when you do indulge in a favorite food, you're riddled with guilt. You find yourself grappling with what you want to eat versus what you believe you should eat.

LEVEL 2: FUNCTIONAL EATING

Your food intake fundamentally meets your needs, even if your food choices seem a bit compromised sometimes. You may not always get to eat sitting down, due to time demands. But all in all, you feel pretty good about your eating habits, your health, your weight, and the amount of energy you have. And even when you can't quite get the food you may want all the time, or you crave a piece of chocolate fudge cake, you don't feel too bent out of shape. You realize it's all going to work out in the end, and you're confident that desserts and other treats, which a lot of people classify as "bad," can be enjoyed in moderation.

You really are an independent eater.

LEVEL 1: OPTIMAL EATING

Your food intake ideally meets your needs. You eat what you want, are capable of balancing your food intake with your energy needs; your food provides your body with optimum nutrition; and no matter where you are, you're able to enjoy eating really well. Either you have enough time to prepare the food you want, or it's prepared properly for you. In short, you celebrate the physical, physiological, mental, and emotional well-being that eating well can bring.

Now, the truth is, most of us have at least visited this level, even if for just the briefest period, but few of us can stay here all the time. The stresses and strains of real life interfere.

In examining your particular food beliefs and food behaviors, you'll undoubtedly see yourself represented on more than one level. And in fact, these levels may relate to different times of your life. You know yourself that when life is going great, it's much easier to eat well. And when time is short, when you're overly stressed, overworked, lonely, unhappy in a relationship or job, that good food habits are often one of the first things to go by the wayside.

What I hope you'll gain out of reading this section is an understanding of what it means to eat well—that is, functionally—no matter what other stuff may be going on in your life. Because in truth, it's when things aren't going well that it's even more important to take the time to eat well. Stressful and difficult times tax our bodies and spirits that much more, so we need to be effectively fueled and emotionally supported by that most essential of substances—food.

FUNCTIONAL FOOD SYSTEMS: A MODEL OF FOOD BEHAVIOR LEADING TO OPTIMAL EATING

Level 5: Out-of-Control Eating

- Eating feels chaotic and out of control—or NOT eating (starvation) is a way to avoid chaos and a sense of being out of control.
- Eating/starving is the way the person copes with life.
- Eating has no connection to hunger or satiety.

Level 4: Rigidly Controlled Eating

- Desperate attempt to control eating behavior.
- Food is controlled with a specific diet plan and/or specific foods.
- One feels either in total control or slips to Level 5 and feels in total chaos.
- Control is the most important issue.
- Sometimes the security of a controlled, structured eating plan is needed before someone can develop more functional and independent ways to eat.

Level 3: Eating by the Rules

- General belief that there is one right way to eat.
- Foods are categorized as "good" or "bad."
- Eating "right" is more important than eating what one wants to eat.
- Eating "bad" foods is considered "cheating."
- Varying levels of guilt are felt when the rules are broken.

Level 2: Functional Eating

- Food choices are made with confidence, and you know you can meet your body's needs.
- Food choices consider your physiological, physical, mental, and emotional needs.
- One manages difficult food situations optimistically—there is a workable solution.
- Sometimes food intake is not its best, but it works for the moment.

Level 1: Optimal Eating

- Food choices are made with confidence, and you know you can meet your body's needs.
- Food choices consider your physiological, physical, mental, and emotional needs.
- There is time and opportunity to make food choices and enjoy eating.

Adapted from Functional Food Systems © 1996 Bonnie Modugno, M.S., R.D.

MOVING THROUGH THE LEVELS TO OPTIMAL EATING

I'm going to describe the process from the bottom, so that you can see how to move up the ladder from out-of-control to optimal eating.

Each step up the ladder—moving from, say, step five to step four, or from step four to step three—represents real developmental progress in food beliefs and food behaviors. In order to help you make that progress, each level has a specific task.

Moving from Out-of-Control to Rigidly Controlled Eating

The most critical skill here is learning to distinguish between true hunger and satiety (that sense of satisfaction you get from eating, not overeating, a wonderful meal). Obviously, if you're stuck in Level 5, overwhelmed by food chaos, this skill may seem as attainable as reaching the summit of Mt. Everest on a skateboard. But it's important to start working with your body and its needs, not against them. Knowing when you're hungry, and when you've had enough, are the most basic cues that lead to independent eating.

It's in Level 5 that you most need support; that support may or may not be a structured food plan. Use the menus provided in order to give your food choices a firm foundation in nutrient balance and moderation. Eat the recommended foods and try to notice how you feel before, while, and after you eat.

It may be tough at first to figure out consciously how you feel; feelings may seem to be all jumbled together in one big tangled mass. But keep at it. You'll be surprised at how quickly the messages your body is sending, that you previously couldn't hear, go from faint whispers to clear messages.

Shortly enough, conscious attention to your feelings will help you to recognize when you feel satisfied, since typically at Level 5 it's tough to discern the difference between when you're hungry and when you've had enough.

One exercise I know that gets great results is choosing to eat only part of the food on your plate. Whether you're at home or at a restaurant, pretend that the last few or several bites aren't there at all. Give yourself ten minutes or so to let what food you've eaten settle, then ask yourself if you're satisfied yet and whether you actu-ally want the remaining portion. What a lot of people don't under-stand is that the stomach's signal to the brain indicating that it's full lags several minutes behind swallowing. So if you are indeed satisfied, then you've learned a valuable lesson: your body didn't need as much as you thought, so now it doesn't have to store those excess calories as fat.

But if the answer is that you're not yet full, then go ahead and eat more. Be sure, though, to distinguish between eating the food out of habit, just because it's there, and eating out of authentic hunger.

Remember, it's especially important to avoid getting overhun-gry, because overhungry people are especially prone to overeating. What you're after here is the ability to stay conscious about when you're hungry and when you're satisfied. Staying focused on that and becoming aware of it means you're making progress.

Moving from Rigidly Controlled to Eating by the Rules

While you may have sense of "enough is enough" now, you're prob-ably still hoping someone will tell you exactly what to eat—even though it's a fact that if you did indeed have a food master lording over your food choices, you'd get sick to death of that person's rein-ing you in all the time. It's human nature to rebel against that. That's why the challenge facing you at this important level is learning what works best for you, and letting the "food police" meddle in someone else's dining room.

That said, it is critical at this level for you to take what you learned about nutrients and build on your new ability to listen to your body's food-related signals. You'll soon learn to determine whether a higher carbohydrate food pattern works for you, or maybe one that contains a little more fat and protein. The focus here is on food composition—the balance of carbohydrates, pro-tein, and fat in your diet.

Remember, everyone is different, made so by genetics, disposi-tion, and environment.

You know that many people are genetically predisposed to insulin resistance; their bodies can't readily convert carbohydrates into glucose. Medical estimates are that one in four normal weight people may be predisposed to insulin resistance. All it takes for them to develop symptoms are the right environmental factors. Meanwhile, even those who aren't otherwise genetically predisposed to insulin resistance risk developing it anyway by gaining too much weight.

If you have not yet figured out which food pattern works best for you, refer back to the section on Food Composition. Review the information, then begin to experiment with the combination of nutrients to find what works best for you.

As before, when you try these different food patterns, pay close attention to how you feel after eating, as well as how long you feel satisfied. Note any differences in how your body looks, or how you feel. Again, I recommend keeping a diary that records your observations after every meal, week to week; they'll lead you to a much clearer and easier understanding of which food patterns work better for you in the overall scheme. And that insight will prove invaluable as you continue making more and better functional food choices while moving up the ladder.

Moving from Eating by the Rules to Functional Eating

Graduating from Level 3 to Level 2 eating is probably the most challenging move of all. Because now comes the time to test your limits and your boundaries.

The point of functional eating is to let go of the rules about what you can eat, what you should eat, how you should eat, when you should eat. Yes, letting go may seem like you've abandoned your lifeline; it's scary and feels risky. But what you have to realize is that *all* growth, *all* risk-taking is scary.

Most everyone listens to different voices in their minds—the voices of teachers, parents, siblings, etc. It's part of living. All the lessons we've ever learned, or tried to learn, join in a chorus that sings in the guise of conscience.

No less developed or acute is that area of conscience devoted to food. Each time we pick up a restaurant menu, walk down a supermarket's aisles, or browse through the refrigerator, somewhere, faintly audible from the depths of the brain, comes the "You shouldn't eat that" or "You should eat this" voice. The outcome of the struggle between the two decides what we buy and eat.

Well, I'd like you to do your best to ignore all those voices. The name of the game here is accountability. At this level you no longer blame experts, diet plans, or your own rules for what doesn't work in your food choices. Your goal is to realize that, for better or worse, you're in charge of choosing your foods. And only you can be accountable for those choices.

Several steps are involved at this stage. First, you have to identify those foods that you consider "good" and "bad." That shouldn't be hard.

Start by dividing a sheet of paper into five columns. Your first column should be titled **Good Food**; the second, **Bad Food**; the third, **Reason**; the fourth, **Foods I Like**; the fifth, **Foods I Dislike**.

Fill up the first three columns with entries. Maybe you think steak is bad because it has too much fat, or broccoli is good because it has a lot of fiber. Maybe you think all sugar and fast foods are bad, and all fruit is good. Just write them down and, in the Reason column add a brief description of why you think they're good or bad.

Fill the last two columns—Like and Dislike. Then notice how many foods you really like that are in the Bad column, and how many are in the Good column. In the same way, compare the foods you dislike.

As you compare, realize that the more often you avoid foods you really like because they're on the Bad list, the more unsatisfied you're likely to be with your current food choices. Not allowing yourself to eat what you like typically translates into a feeling of deprivation and dissatisfaction—and ultimately resentment.

By the same token, if you eat foods you dislike only because they're supposed to be "good for you," you're more likely to rebel against your food choices. If you don't feel it now, you eventually will.

Like most people, you probably believe that french fries are a taboo food. Conventional wisdom says that you should stay away from them . . . because they're fried. And yet, eating french fries with a skinless chicken breast and some steamed vegetables may be just the balance of fat, protein, and carbohydrate that leaves you feeling perfectly satisfied. That same meal without the fries could leave you unsatisfied and feeling deprived—so you'll return over and over to the refrigerator or cupboard all night looking for a way to fill that hole. I'd say most people get into trouble at some time or another by snacking all night long after leaving the dinner table dissatisfied.

In fact, there's no way to state categorically that there are "good" foods and "bad" foods. Sure, the foods on your Good list are probably terrific. But I'm sure a good case can be made that any of those Bad list foods are equally functional, depending on circumstances.

If that's true for french fries, doesn't it follow then that the other foods on your bad list—pizza, candy, tacos, cheese, butter, etc.— may also find comfortable niches in your diet? Whether or not a food is functional depends on your body, your (weight loss) goals, your circumstances, and the food's place in the rest of your diet.

As you move toward developing the more functional food choices of Level 2, you have an opportunity to restructure your approach to food, the way you think about it.

The goal at this stage is to begin including some of the foods you like best into your food plan. In every meal, eat something you really yearn for but which you've rarely in the past allowed yourself to eat—at least not without guilt. Now, though, I want you to eat that food in balance with the other foods in your meal. Do it and notice what happens. If occasionally the item is a dessert, make sure to eat a balanced meal first, stopping just short of satiety so that you have adequate room—and vibrant tastebuds—for your chocolate cake, or mud pie, or whatever.

By "saving room" for that treat after eating a reasonable meal, you may find that a few bites of it is enough. But if it's not enough, don't worry. This is a great time to satisfy your desire for that special something else. Enjoy it!

One final word about this level. If you ever find yourself really splurging—that is, going overboard; feeling out of control at a certain meal—don't be too hard on yourself. A single meal, no matter how badly you think you've overeaten, or how full you feel, is not a disaster. As long as you keep that episode unique and don't tumble into a pattern of continued overeating, the extra weight you may notice the next morning will disappear in a few days. You'll metabolize those calories, and you can be back on track with your very next meal.

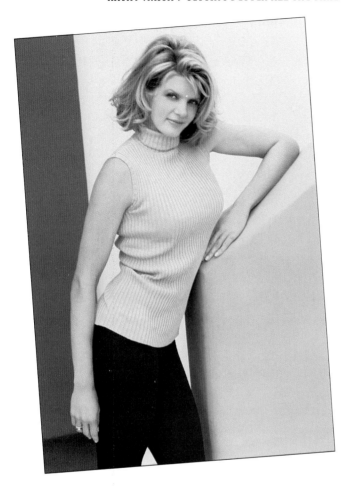

Moving from Functional Eating to Optimal Eating

Let me be completely honest: Eating consistently at Level 1 is tough for most people who aren't on permanent vacation. Because if you keep an ordinary, busy schedule, you probably don't have the time or energy to do what's necessary. Myself included. I can be a Level 1 eater when my schedule permits. Then I have the time to prepare food properly and relax enough to enjoy all the pleasure food provides. I don't have to worry about endless "To Do" lists. I don't have to rush from meeting to meeting.

Yes, I would prefer to eat at Level 1 all the time. But, like you, I live in the real world—and it's a busy world. This is where Level 2 eating works just fine, thank you. I don't beat myself up when I can't stay at Level 1. I just accept the ebb and flow of the process, and utterly savor those times when Level 1 is achievable.

A PERSPECTIVE ON THE PROCESS

It would be wonderful if reading this book settles, once and for all, your food-related issues. But managing your food choices is an ongoing process, it's part of the idea of *Getting Better All the Time*. Sometimes choices will be automatic, almost mindless. Other times you'll struggle. This is when you need to pay more attention, using all your problem-solving skills.

At the least, I hope that exposing you to new kinds of thinking, planning, and experimenting with foods will improve your attitude about food and help you to learn to enjoy food's rightful place in your life. Ideally, I'd like you to spend most of your eating time enjoying the flexibility and choices of Level 1 and Level 2. But I'd also like you not to beat yourself up as you're working to move forward from more troublesome eating patterns, or despair once you achieve more independent eating and occasionally slip to Levels 3, 4, or 5.

Please understand that everyone slips from time to time. The experience you get from working your way up the ladder through the levels is bound to give you that much more confidence and reinforcement when you return again to functional eating patterns; you'll have a broader perspective and point of view. As in many other areas of life, you can probably learn more from slipping up than you can from success. Of course, enjoying more functional eating remains your ultimate goal.

You achieve success—that is, climb the ladder back to Levels 1 and 2—by choosing better food options as a response to each time you slip. Allow yourself the time and space to figure out what may have caused the slip, then mentally rehearse choosing a better option the next time you're presented with a similar challenge. That's how you build a storehouse of food options and strategies to meet any situation. It allows you to stay in true control of your food and your eating through choice and flexibility.

To get a better idea of how the process works, take a look at the following model.

A MODEL OF PROBLEM SOLVING

PROBLEM: Identify the specific issue to be addressed.

EXAMPLE: *"I keep overeating every evening after dinner because I don't feel satisfied."*

OPTIONS: Brainstorm and identify possible options for this particular problem. You could, for example:

Option 1. "Keep eating until I feel full."

Option 2. "Check to see if I ate adequate fat and/or protein in my meal to feel satisfied."

Option 3. "Look at the whole day's food intake. Did I eat too little during the day and got overhungry so I needed to overeat?"

Option 4. "Did I really just want a piece of chocolate—but tried to 'be good' by eating too much of everything else?"

SOLUTION: Choose an option and test it out:

"I skipped lunch so I could leave early and pick up my kids before six o'clock. I don't think I ate enough all day long. So maybe next time I'll eat a sandwich and yogurt at my desk and give myself a late afternoon snack so I don't feel so ravenous at night."

EVALUATION: Look at your results and decide if you've hit on a good solution, or whether you need to keep looking:

"I felt a lot better. I wasn't crabby through the afternoon, and after dinner I felt more content." (Wonderful! This option worked.)

Or: "I still want something sweet after dinner. What's wrong with me? But I have to admit I didn't overeat as much." (Good start! You solved part of your problem, now take this smaller problem and run it through the process again.)

YOUR METABOLISM

As you're working with these food plans, it's important to be aware of some general concepts about metabolism. Much of this may seem obvious, though I've found that it's sometimes easy to miss the simpler issues when we're so fully preoccupied by the challenge of what to eat and how to eat.

This section is about what you can do to keep your metabolism at its highest level through eating properly. The first message here is, don't skip meals, especially "breakfast"—or whatever you choose to eat for your first meal of the day.

There are a thousand excuses for skipping breakfast, inadequate time being number one. But there's only one good reason to make time for what the old saying correctly notes is "the most important meal of the day": Skipping it—or calling a quick glass of juice or coffee breakfast—sends unpleasant and unintended shock waves through the day, while a good breakfast helps your system hum.

Eating earlier in the day kicks your metabolism into a higher gear. Ironically, your body actually makes it easy to skip this important meal, because whenever you fast for a period of time (while you were sleeping, in this case) your body taps into some of the calories from your meal last night that were stored as glycogen. You may remember that glycogen is a carbohydrate that rapidly breaks down to glucose, the blood sugar that all cells use for energy. So until that store is used up, you can easily fight those hunger pangs, knowing that in a few minutes they'll go away—because a body that's not fed when it's hungry will initiate a series of biochemical reactions, resulting in the liver's releasing some of the stored glycogen into the blood. As blood sugar rises, hunger is calmed (as long as there is stored glycogen).

But not without consequences.

The difference between eating to raise your blood sugar and not eating to raise your blood sugar can be profound. That stored glycogen doesn't last all day, and when it runs out, you typically go directly from hungry to overhungry without passing Go.

No matter where I'm hiking around the world, I always make time to check in with the girls.

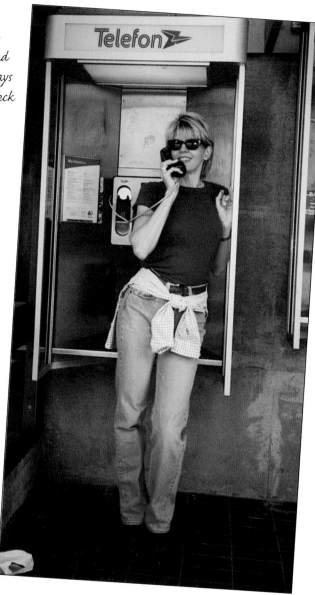

Overhungry typically leads to overeating—many times, all night long.

Even more devastating, though, is what kind of message this sort of eating gives your body: It tells your body that you're starving. And a starving body slows its metabolism down to survive.

EAT ENOUGH CALORIES: Generally speaking, it takes some pretty sophisticated equipment to determine how many calories someone needs a day. So I can't pretend to know what your individual caloric needs are. You, however, probably have a good sense of whether you have a "slow metabolism" or a fast one. If you think you have a slow metabolism, maybe it's because: 1) you have been restricting your calories severely in order to lose weight; 2) you may have inadvertently taught your body to prepare for starvation (as in eating too little all day long or on into the night); 3) you are chronically dieting; or 4) you have instigated a loss of muscle mass with either chronic dieting or lack of exercise.

The body has evolved over thousands of years in which famine, drought, and trauma were the norms. It stores fat weight like a squirrel preparing for winter. Hungry for nourishment, it hoards calories when it gets them; it doesn't burn them. But in late twentieth-century America, famine and drought are not the problems they were. So you may need to actually increase your calorie intake to assume a more normal metabolic rate before you can expect to see fat loss, if that's your goal. Only then will it react to the program as intended.

Try introducing slightly larger amounts of food into your diet gradually, while engaging in regular physical activity. Any exercise will help your body rebuild muscle mass that broke down when you were restricting your calories, but weight training is especially effective. And you want to rebuild muscle mass because it's among the body's most metabolically active tissues, which means that, as a rule, the more muscle you have, the higher your metabolic rate.

In the meantime, if you happen to gain a few pounds during this transition period, don't get too anxious. It's probably muscle weight, and when your metabolic rate picks up again, you'll be able to metabolize these additional calories, as well as feel stronger and more satisfied.

At this point, I should add that for some people, whose weight and eating problems are extreme, this process may be too daunting to tackle alone. They may need professional help, someone to whom they can turn for psychological advice and emotional support or nutritional guidance. I've listed resources in the Nutrition Appendix on page 186.

If you think your metabolism falls in the normal range, let your hunger and satiety be your guide. Once you find a food composition that works well for you, you'll be able to listen to your body, and trust what it tells you.

PHYSICAL ACTIVITY AND METABOLISM: Physically active bodies produce more of the enzymes that are needed to convert fat into fuel. So a fit person can metabolize and lose fat weight much more readily than someone who is out of shape.

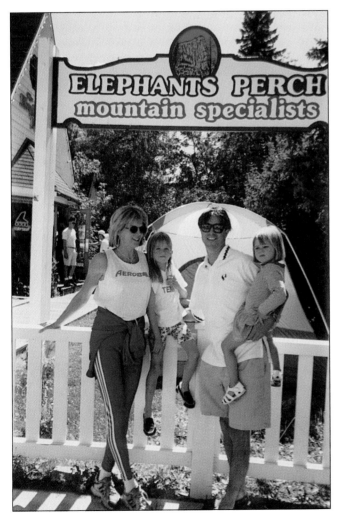

One of our favorite vacation spots is Sun Valley, where we can spend time together hiking and camping.

What's more, with that greater access to fat, the body doesn't have to rely as much on glucose for fuel—a distinct advantage for weight management. When you use more fat for fuel, as opposed to glucose for fuel, you won't feel excessively hungry after exercise. But if you do get light-headed, shaky, and weak after working out, you probably need more calories—or maybe more protein and fat—in your diet. (See earlier section on Food Composition.) If you are ready for a meal, this is a good time to eat, because the muscles store glycogen from carbohydrates most efficiently 1 to 2 hours after a workout.

Another huge advantage of exercise is your body's increased sensitivity to insulin (the opposite of insulin resistance), which means you'll be able to use carbohydrates more effectively.

Physical activity also allows you to increase your lean body mass, which is comprised of bone, blood, vital organs, and muscle tissue. The more muscle you have, the higher your metabolic rate. Increasing your lean body mass, along with adequate caloric intake, are the most significant actions you can take to improve your metabolic rate.

Studies show that, contrary to what we've always believed, a slowed metabolism doesn't have to accompany the aging process; it can run at practically the same rate by maintaining lean body mass. But it's easy to see why we've thought the two go hand in hand: Since senior citizens in the past became less active over the years, they lost their lean body mass, and so it followed that their metabolisms slowed. But researchers now agree that the elderly can build muscle mass and increase their metabolism at any age, by working out aerobically and with weights. Bottom line: it's never too late.

At every age, physical activity is critically important. The important thing to remember is that a fit person can enjoy a stronger metabolism, burn fat better, and have more energy than an unfit person.

WHEN SHOULD I EAT?: For years, the biggest myth about when to eat was that you shouldn't eat after 6:00 P.M. There are also many guilt-producing rules, such as "three square meals a day," "six smaller meals a day," "No snacking between meals," etc.

Truth is, no one way to eat is best for everyone. What's best for you may not be found until you experiment.

Depending on your preferences, you may want to snack often and eat smaller meals, or you may want to have those three squares a day with nothing in between. It's funny, but having the freedom to experiment will probably connect you better to your own hunger, enabling you to decide what and how much to eat.

If you find yourself consuming most of your food just before bedtime, you are courting fat storage. If you're active enough and use the fat stores for energy the next day, you'll probably manage your weight just fine. But if you're not active enough to do that, the fat will continue to accumulate over time.

Try thinking about your day in sections, throughout your waking hours—and fuel your body accordingly for each section. This is especially important for people who work atypical hours. Your goal: to eat as your body needs fuel and avoid getting overhungry. If this means three times a day, great. If it means six times a day, that's fine, too. As you know, getting overhungry means you're likely to overeat. There's no such thing as saving calories for later; it only causes more problems than it's worth. Not only do you feel less than your best when overhungry, you're certainly not going to feel that great after overeating later.

FOOD: ACCESS AND AVAILABILITY: The basic issue in whether you have access to good food is time—time to purchase it, time to prepare it, time to chew it, time to swallow it. Time comes into play whether we eat at home or out. Time (and money) can determine what we eat, how we eat, and whether we enjoy what we're eating. Not having enough time usually translates into settling for mediocre food, or eating too fast, too much, or not at all. So you can see that when it comes to eating well, inadequate time compromises a lot more than just the food.

Think of how you react to the stresses of time. Maybe you think that you don't have time to eat a proper breakfast or lunch, so you get overhungry and then later on eat whatever happens to be around. But whether it's an apple or a candy bar, it's still not adequate.

Maybe you feel pressured with too much to do, so you end up

skipping a meal. And you get a headache, feel irritable, or have difficulty concentrating well—and spend twice as much time doing the very thing you wanted to get over with quickly anyway. Why? Because your brain is starving. It's screaming, "Feed me."

All of which is to say that if you're serious about taking care of yourself and making good choices in life, you need to consider better when and how you eat.

GETTING FOOD: Two questions here: What? and When?

First, what. You have several factors to consider in deciding what to eat. But if you wait until you're hungry, you probably won't have as many choices as you would if you had planned ahead. Getting to the grocery store regularly is the key to keeping the cupboard and refrigerator well-stocked with good foods. If you're not in the habit of shopping on a regular basis, ask yourself why. Your answer will probably be one of the following excuses—since I've heard them all:

- *"I hate shopping."* This is a common one, and usually applies only to food, not clothing. If you don't like to shop for food, then try to muster the strength to find a way through your dislike, or get someone else, maybe a family member, to do it for you. These days, a lot of markets have home delivery, and some will even shop for you.
- *"I don't have time."* Time is the thing most of us have the least of. But the truth is, it takes a lot less time to shop for the week ahead than to figure out what you're going to eat on a meal-by-meal basis. Don't kid yourself; you're eventually going to have to eat, and it's going to take time to get that food.
- *"My schedule is erratic. I can't depend on being home to cook."* These days, with people often working longer hours or two jobs to get by, this is a good, legitimate excuse. But there's still an antidote: Keep staples on hand and use your freezer. Frozen foods are a lot more nutritious than anything that rots in your refrigerator and never gets eaten anyway. A few choice canned and packaged foods can at least get you by for that occasional meal at home.

- *"I don't know how"* or *"I feel overwhelmed."* In this day and age, food shopping and food preparation are fast becoming lost arts. Too many of us grow up without learning how. So ask someone to go to the market with you. A friend, a relative, maybe a coworker. Be honest about your dilemma and ask for help. You'll be surprised at how willing others will be to assist you—including the store personnel. All it takes is once or twice and you'll be a whiz with that shopping cart.
- *"I eat most of my meals out."* Fine. This means your needs are fewer than most. You'll probably need only a handful of foods for that rare occasion when you're eating home. For you, a couple of cans of soup, tuna, and tomato sauce to go with a package of pasta and some frozen vegetables will be great.
- *"I hate to cook."* Listen, a lot of people hate to cook. But they also like to eat. So if you don't want to eat every meal out, familiarize yourself with the many great foods that supermarkets carry nowadays that take very little preparation. The deli and frozen foods cases are full of them. Ask someone you trust or the store manager to point the way.
- *"I'd rather eat out."* Terrific. Please, enjoy it. Yes, it takes more care to eat healthily, but it's wonderful if you have the time and finances to do it well.
- *"If I buy it, I eat it."* Keeping a small amount of food in the house is an effective food-management technique. Most people benefit if they limit how much candy, sodas, and other snack foods they keep in the house. But if bringing adequate healthy foods into the house feels too scary, you may want to discuss the matter with either a therapist or a nutritionist. (See Nutrition Appendix on page 186 for references.)

Once you've determined how often you want to prepare food in your own home, then get to the market and stock your kitchen with that amount of food. Remember to get the variety of nutrients you need. Choose a variety of carbohydrates from fruits, vegetables, grain products, and proteins from vegetable/animal sources. But also remember to include your favorite sources of fat: oils, nuts, seeds, salad dressing, mayonnaise, margarine and/or butter, etc.

If you're looking for convenience, take advantage of what's available: precut and cleaned lettuce; prepared vegetables that are ready to be steamed, fruit chunks that can be thrown together quickly for a fruit salad; and hot entreés from the deli section. You may find that you need to augment some of those preprepared portions with an extra dish in order to get the right balance of nutrients and calories for you. Try a side salad or bowl of soup, maybe a baked potato if you do better with a high-carbohydrate diet. And if you need additional protein and fat, add some chopped nuts to a salad or some extra clams to your bowl of clam chowder.

I can't think of an excuse in the world why you can't let the convenience of today's wonderful supermarkets work for you.

FOOD PREPARATION: In the world of food preparation, there are two kinds of people: those who know how to cook, and those who don't.

Actually, there may be two other kinds of people, as well: those who like to cook and those who don't.

Come to think of it, there may also be another two: those who have to cook, and those who don't. In my experience, it's rare to find a person who (a) has to cook, (b) knows how to cook, and (c) really likes to cook. But no matter.

The majority of us identify with some mix of these elements; whether we like it or not, we do have to prepare food for ourselves and/or our families at least some of the time. Sadly, cooking is often a thankless task, particularly if you're the only one doing it and you're always playing "Beat the Clock."

If food preparation for you or your family ranks high on your list, then find the time. Take it, if you have to, from something else that ranks lower on the list.

For me, cooking is especially enjoyable when I can include my children. Being in the kitchen together, creating delicious meals, becomes a wonderfully intimate time. Maybe it's because I'm taking the time to teach them these skills. Or maybe it's just the feeling that we're doing this together. Or maybe it's just that we're together, period. We talk, we listen, we chop vegetables, we measure ingredients. The most mundane aspect of cooking seems as though it's been elevated to a higher level. I savor these moments, and because I do I make more time for them—which means more home-cooked meals.

That said, there's nothing wrong with throwing together a meal if you have to. Not every meal has to be worthy of the great chefs of France. Using the best of the convenience items at your local market—prewashed vegetables and fruit, preseasoned and cubed meats and fish—can yield terrifically worthy meals in minutes.

So at one end you have convenience; all that takes is a little planning ahead: having the proper foods there when you need them. At the other end you have the luxury of flipping through cookbooks, targeting a recipe, and taking your sweet time in preparing it. Either choice can serve you well.

EATING OUT: Eating out has become a way of life for most Americans. One of the restaurant trade associations estimates that more than 60 percent of all meals are eaten away from home, and that 42 cents of every food dollar is spent on food prepared away from home.

This makes sense when you consider how busy we've all become over the last decade or so, with many people holding down two jobs or at least working longer hours.

Now, while I suspect that a high percentage of those meals eaten away from home are eaten at fast-food restaurants, the good news is that eating out doesn't have to be a nutritional disaster. Over the past few years, even fast-food places have seen the light and offer a larger variety of choices from their menus, including some healthful food options.

Even so, when I go out to eat, which I do frequently, I don't make myself crazy by paying attention to every single ingredient. In fact, if I want those french fries, I order them. But if I'm feeling a bit concerned that the meal has too much fat, maybe I'll order a chicken breast sandwich instead of a hamburger. The point is, I try not to deprive myself of what I really want to eat, and yet stay accountable for the choices I do make. What I've learned from experience is that if I choose consciously, I'm less likely to regret my choice later.

But then there's the issue of quantity at the restaurant. Some places serve portions that could feed an entire family. Other places set down entrées that look more like finger-food appetizers. So if you don't know the restaurant, you may not know what you're getting when you order. Just ask your server how big the portions are. Ultimately, it's your decision to stop when you've had enough. You can always take the rest home and eat it for lunch tomorrow.

Another issue related to eating out is about "saving up calories" in order to eat out. Don't do it. Please. Because if you do, you'll be overhungry and probably attack the bread basket. So either you'll be stuffed before the entrée arrives or you won't be able to eat slowly enough to enjoy the food, much less pay attention to anything else. It's better that you eat normally through the day, and then enjoy the eating experience when you dine later.

One last word about restaurants. If you decide to indulge, enjoy. A single meal never made anyone fat or permanently raised cholesterol. Notice I said "a single meal." A healthy eating pattern allows for the occasional indulgence.

We live busy, and usually stressful, lives. And we need emotional nurturing, even with food.

But using food as a coping mechanism isn't real nurturing. It only keeps us from resolving whatever issues are really bothering us.

Using food to nurture ourselves emotionally is about recognizing our needs and learning how to use food as a vehicle for meeting those needs. Sometimes when I'm hungry and tired, I just want to feel warm and cuddled. I get that from a bowl of hot, hearty soup. I guess that's why they call it "comfort food."

And sometimes I crave solid food when I'm feeling worn out. That piece of swordfish with a baked potato and salad will hit just the spot.

Other times I need something that's light, cold, refreshing—a crisp salad or fresh fruit with yogurt. And when I decide to enjoy a piece of chocolate, give me the best there is; I want to savor every bite. This is how food can be used to satisfy our emotional needs.

Food is about flavor. It's about texture. Temperature. Color. Presentation. All of those elements work to nurture us. And they do so when we take the time to notice each of them.

In its rightful place, food can be an incredibly satisfying part of our lives. What I hope is that reading my thoughts on the matter

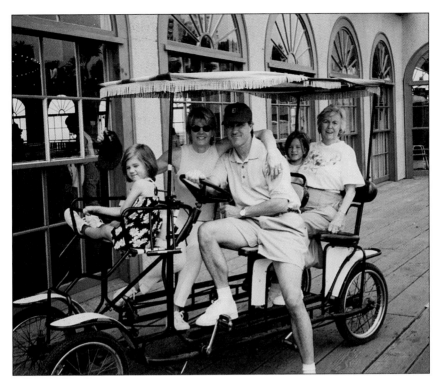

*Santa Monica Pier. The family that plays together stays fit together.
Even Grandma Mimi joins the fun.*

have inspired you and educated you on how to make your best food choices. I'd like food to be both what you want it to be and need it to be. I'd like you to enjoy every bite, secure in the knowledge that what you're eating serves you well.

NUTRITION APPENDIX

If you feel that your food-related issues need greater attention than this (or any) book can provide, you may want to consider calling one of the following numbers for counseling assistance. I encourage you to do so.

American Anorexia/Bulimia Association, Inc.
165 W. 46th Street
Suite 1108
New York, NY 10036
(212) 575-6200

Anorexia Nervosa and Related Eating Disorders, Inc.
P.O. Box 5102
Eugene, Oregon 97405
(541) 344-1144

American Dietetic Association (referral service)
(800) 366-1655

American Psychological Association
(800) 374-2721

Nutrition consultant for this book:

Ms. Bonnie Modugno, M.S., R.D.
530 Wilshire Boulevard
Suite 310
Santa Monica, CA 90401
(310) 395-4822

PART THREE
THE POWER OF FITNESS

CONGRATULATIONS, YOU'RE NOW EQUIPPED WITH VERY powerful information to help motivate you, and to help you make healthy choices about your eating. Now it's time to turn your attention to the final part of my plan—and my favorite topic.

Exercise.

Are you wincing already? I hope not.

Can there be any doubt in your mind about the benefits of exercise? I'm sure you've seen the newspaper, radio, and television reports. Dozens, perhaps even hundreds, of studies in recent years are unanimous in their conclusions: Regular exercise can change your life.

It's obvious that regular exercise will help you maintain a healthy weight. What all the studies have also demonstrated is that exercise can do everything from lowering your risk of heart disease, to easing the symptoms of menstruation. It has been associated with a dramatic decline in depression and is a factor in decreasing hypertension. The simple truth is, exercise works.

If you agree with that premise, then the only question at this point can be: How do you get started, and maintain, a regular exercise plan?

Well, guess what? That's just what my Power of Choice Fitness Plan will do.

The program focuses on the three key areas of exercise:

- cardiovascular or "aerobic" exercise
- strength training
- flexibility (stretching and relaxation)

Working each of these components is essential. You can't just focus on an aerobic activity and avoid strengthening your muscles. The same holds true for flexibility. The body just doesn't work that way.

But trust me, my program is not overly rigid. Each part of it is designed to give you choices. For example, in the cardiovascular section you can choose any aerobic activity you like—from aerobics classes to swimming, from mountain biking to jogging. Or if you prefer a set regimen, I've designed a really neat, all-inclusive walking program, one that meets your cardiovascular requirements.

Strength training is the second essential area of my exercise plan. The approach is designed to take the mystery (and fear) out of building muscles. Please don't get hung up on stereotypes of muscle-bound men and women. When you read the strength section, you'll immediately appreciate the benefits of building stronger muscles.

The third key area is flexibility. I wouldn't consider this an area people fear; rather, they just don't understand it. So maybe you'll be surprised to hear that it's the most important of the three categories. Without flexibility, simple daily activities—such as bending, twisting, getting out of your car—become a challenge. Flexibility through stretching and relaxation even pays off in stress reduction. This is the area of exercise where I make a mind and body connection. If you trust me and work in this area, you'll witness significant life changes with regular flexibility exercise.

Finally, what I think is the most special aspect of my plan: it's devised around a concept called "periodization." While this word is probably unfamiliar to you, trust me, periodization will help you overcome any exercise obstacle.

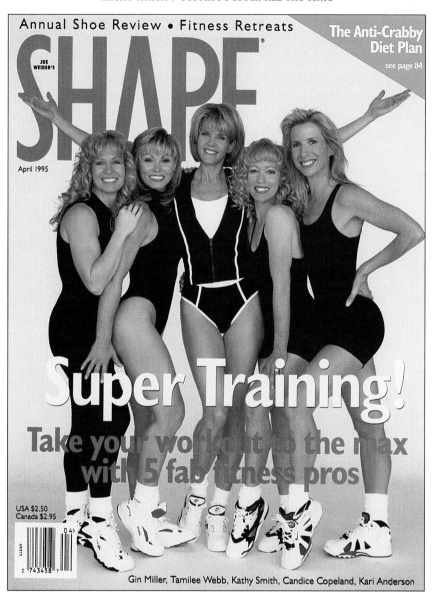

Annual Shoe Review • Fitness Retreats

The Anti-Crabby Diet Plan
see page 84

JOE WEIDER'S

SHAPE®

April 1995

Super Training!
Take your workout to the max with 5 fab fitness pros

USA $2.50
Canada $2.95

Gin Miller, Tamilee Webb, Kathy Smith, Candice Copeland, Kari Anderson

Shape magazine, 1995.

In simple terms, periodization refers to choice, helping you vary the type of workout and the intensity of your workout. This method is used by elite athletes to motivate them, and to help prevent boredom. And it's a concept that's missing in nearly every exercise program out there today.

I've designed my Power of Choice program with all fitness levels in mind. I've included a six-week periodization plan as part of your fitness routine that will help you maximize your results. Most important, it's a fitness program for life. So as you progress, you'll be able to make choices and changes all along the way.

According to a recent poll, more than 70 of America's top 100 CEOs schedule at least three hours a week of exercise into their incredibly busy schedules. That tells us a lot. These are very successful men and women who rise early every morning, get to the gym for a brisk workout, have breakfast, then go to the office for probably twelve hours. Now, they could be exercising for nothing more than stress reduction, considering how stressful running billion-dollar companies must be. Or, they could be working out because fitness helps them in their business lives. (I know it helps me; between deadlines and heavy workloads, I sometimes have to call upon stamina that wouldn't be there if not for my fitness level.) Or they could be working out because they need some fun and recreation—period. Or they want to look and feel better, knowing what a competitive advantage that gives them. For whatever reason they work out, the fact that they do it at all just helps to prove that good health and fitness are connected to success. These CEOs must have found something powerful in this thing called exercise.

Even if you've never in your life done anything that could remotely be called exercise, you can begin turning the tide by starting a regular program. Every month, it seems, there's a new study about the benefits of exercise. The one that may have had the greatest impact on me was the one that studied nursing home residents, ages eighty-six to ninety. The participants were started on a vigorous exercise program, including lifting weights. In just eight weeks, they increased their strength by 175 percent. Two of them actually threw away their canes.

After the strength program, these people were then put on fitness programs, in order to increase their cardiovascular capabilities. Almost every one of them reported dramatic gains in overall quality of life. (One study I read concluded that elderly people who began an exercise program greatly improved their powers of concentration and memory.) So the good news is, it's never too late to begin, no matter how old you are.

Right now, you can begin taking steps to slow down the aging process. Many of the problems we once thought of as being inevitably related to the aging process aren't necessarily going to arise, especially if you're involved in a fitness program and stick to it. My Power of Choice Fitness Plan, which includes cardiovascular, strength, and flexibility training, is just that kind of program.

It never ceases to amaze me how exercise can benefit every aspect of our health. Here's a list of what increases or goes up when you exercise:

WHAT GOES UP

muscle tone
heart strength
cardiac blood volume
oxygen uptake
bone strength
lung function
ability to sleep well
mental fitness
"good" cholesterol
resistance to colds and flu
immune system
red blood cell production
blood volume
circulation
self-esteem
energy level
digestion
improved balance

Conversely, here's a list of what decreases or goes down with regular exercise:

WHAT GOES DOWN

body fat
weight
stress
appetite
blood pressure
resting pulse
cardiovascular disease
gallbladder disease
"bad" cholesterol
diabetes risk
colon cancer risk
varicose veins
constipation
depression

All these benefits and yet only about two in ten adults perform some type of regular athletic activity—and 50 percent(!) are completely sedentary. Do they know what they're missing? Maybe, maybe not. Or maybe they're members of a growing club: the half of all people who start an exercise program but quit within six months. Many of them even pay for the privilege: nearly four out of ten people who join health clubs drop out each year.

You can be sure that all of those people who dropped out or quit had good intentions; they wanted to be fit and knew they had to work out in order to get fit. A recent national survey showed that about 90 percent of Americans understand that exercise is something they should be doing.

The problem is, most people just don't stick with their programs. Why not? Everyone has a different excuse.

SO WHAT'S YOUR EXCUSE?

Let's focus on some of the most common excuses for not exercising. Look at the following excuses and see whether some of my solutions can help. If not, you may want to refer back to Brainstorm Solutions (page 33) in order to solve your particular problem.

"I HAVE NO TIME TO EXERCISE."

This is the excuse I hear most often. I empathize with it because I have the exact same problem. Here are some suggestions to try to find time in your day:

1. Get up earlier two mornings a week.

2. Ask your spouse/significant other to help with dinner or dishes two days a week, so that you can work out.

3. Meet a friend after work, or at the end of the day, for a workout. You'll get a chance to socialize and keep each other motivated.

4. Work out to a favorite TV show. If it happens to be on at a time that's inconvenient to exercise, tape it and save it for a workout. (I like to do this with *Frasier.*)

5. Exercise is cumulative, so dividing your workout into two parts—some in the morning, some in the evening—is just as good as doing it in one session.

6. Grab a walk during your lunch break.

"I'M TOO TIRED TO EXERCISE."

1. This is one reason I don't exercise at the end of the day. I exercise in the mornings because it's when my energy is at its peak. The day's events haven't yet started to interfere.

2. Make sure you're getting enough sleep.

3. Shift your mind-set (refer back to Shift Your Mind-set, page 44). Instead of focusing on how tired you are, choose to focus on how good you'll feel after working out.

4. I've found that having a ritual sometimes helps to get you in the mood, particularly when fatigue is a factor. I make myself a vitamin C drink, start chewing on a piece of bubble gum, then lie on

the floor, press my hips up in the air, so I get a little blood flowing to my head. Finally, I take some deep breaths . . . and I feel energized.

"EXERCISING BORES ME."

This one's a little hard for me to understand. There are so many options and choices—as you'll see when you begin the Power of Choice Fitness Plan.

1. Close your eyes and remember a time when you were in grade school, sitting at your desk, praying for the recess bell to ring. You ran to the playground, alive with the anticipation of playing. Playing what?

2. Change your mind-set. Stop thinking of it as drudgery. Think of it as time for yourself.

3. Fantasize while working out. My favorite fantasy is to imagine myself as a rock star, driving 65,000 people into a frenzy with my extraordinary talent. (If you've ever heard me sing, you'd realize what a real fantasy this is.)

"I DIDN'T GET THE RESULTS I WANTED, SO I GAVE UP."

Not getting results can be discouraging. But when you look over the list of exercise benefits beginning on page 191, you'll see there's no such thing as "not getting results."

While you may not have gotten down to your target weight as quickly as you would have liked, you're still affecting every system in your body. You're doing yourself an awful lot of good, even if it doesn't seem like it.

"EXERCISING IS TOO EXPENSIVE."

An exercise program doesn't have to be expensive. All you need is a pair of workout shoes and some dumbbells.

1. Keep your eyes open at garage sales for used dumbbells.

2. Put the cost of dumbbells in perspective. What is their real cost measured against the enormous benefits you'll do yourself? As the old saying goes: "An ounce of prevention is worth a pound of cure."

3. Dumbbells aren't much more expensive than a few manicures or movies.

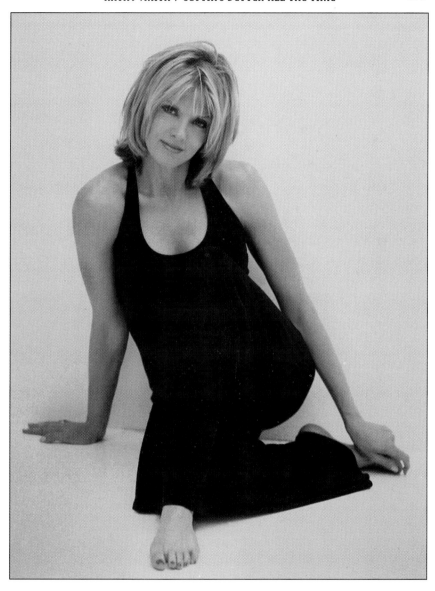

WHICH ACTIVITIES ARE RIGHT FOR YOU?

Even people who understand the benefits of exercise, and are motivated to do it, often abandon their exercise program. Why? Because they choose programs they think they *ought* to do but don't enjoy. In my Power of Choice Fitness Plan, on the other hand, you'll be choosing activities you enjoy and will therefore be more likely to stick with.

Let me give you an example. I have a friend named Lisa who's in terrific shape. She wakes early every morning and runs four miles before work. One of her coworkers, Tina, became so impressed by the great shape Lisa is in, she decided she'd copy Lisa's program. To her, it made sense: Lisa looks great, I want to look like Lisa; so I'll do what Lisa does. Every morning Tina awoke, laced up her new running shoes, and hit the highway for a four-mile jog. Trouble was, Tina didn't like to run; in fact, she'd always hated it. Not only that, but she truly disliked the time alone; she preferred company. Plus, she'd never been a morning person in her life. Her body rhythms seemed to be set for the p.m. hours, especially for strenuous activities—which had never included running, anyway.

So, of course, Tina managed to struggle through the routine for only four weeks. When she gave up (with a sigh of relief), she decided that she and exercise were incompatible and that she would never look as fit as Lisa.

This story represents so many people out there.

Exercise has to fit who you are every bit as well as your clothes do. Doing it shouldn't be a daily struggle.

When you choose exercises that fit you, there's no struggle involved; they mold easily into your lifestyle.

The bottom line: you don't have to think of exercise as that thing you do only at the gym or on the track. The truth is, any activity that gets you moving (regularly) is exercise.

YOUR PERSONAL EXERCISE PROFILE

Evaluate your lifestyle in order to choose your exercise activities wisely. The answers to these six questions will help you.

1. Do you like to exercise alone or with friends?
2. Does morning or evening exercise fit your body rhythm or schedule better?
3. Does music help motivate you?
4. What activities do you enjoy doing?
5. What activities did you enjoy doing as a child?
6. What are your hobbies?

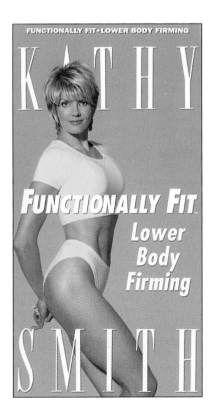

This was my twenty-second video. At forty-five years old I feel better than I did when I first started making videos. "Getting Better All the Time!"

Tina remembered that as a child she used to dance a lot. She loved being out there at parties, listening to the music, being with friends—in other words, making it a social situation.

I suggested that she join a club where she could take a dance movement class. That sounded great to her. She called around to several clubs until she found one that offered this kind of class that would fit her schedule. Now, more than a year later, she still goes three nights a week to her hour-long class, and loves every minute of it, she says—so much so that she claims not to have missed more than four classes total the entire year. She's as fit as she wants to be and happy with the results.

The moral of Tina's story is that wrong choices make for bad exercise experiences, while good ones lead to consistency . . . which leads to fitness.

Exercise comes in many forms. The idea is to get your body moving and burn calories—in other words, to get you off the couch and into motion. With so many choices available, you're sure to find one that fits your personal exercise profile.

Take a look at the chart on the next page to see where your favorite activity rates by calories burned.

These are all great activities for calorie-burning even though they vary in terms of intensity. I hope there's something on this chart that tickles your fancy, and I want you to consider this: walking moderately burns eighty-eight calories in fifteen minutes. That's pretty good. But gardening, believe it or not, burns about sixty calories in the same fifteen minutes. And if you add in some raking during that time, you're probably burning as many calories as if you did walking, while at the same time getting something done that you either like to do or maybe had to do anyway.

CALORIES BURNED

ACTIVITY	MINUTES			
	15	**30**	**45**	**60**
Aerobics (high impact)	104	207	311	414
Aerobics (low impact)	74	148	222	296
Ballet	89	177	266	354
Bicycling (12–14 mph)	118	236	354	472
Box aerobics	133	265	398	530
Circuit weight training	118	236	354	472
Cross-country skiing	150	300	450	600
Downhill skiing	74	148	222	296
Golf (carrying clubs)	81	162	243	324
In-line skating	104	207	311	414
Jumping rope (moderate)	148	295	443	590
Karate, tae kwon do	148	295	443	590
Kayaking	74	148	222	296
Mountain biking	126	251	377	502
Racquetball	104	207	311	414
Rowing machine	150	300	450	600
Running (8.5-min. mile)	170	339	509	678
Ski machine	140	280	320	560
Slide (moderate)	101	201	302	402
Stairclimber	105	210	315	420
Stationary bike (vigorous)	155	310	465	620
Step aerobics	169	337	506	674
Swimming (crawl, 50 yd./min.)	143	285	428	570
Tai chi	59	118	177	236
Tennis (singles)	118	236	354	472
VersaClimber	161	322	483	644
Walking (12-min. mile)	113	225	413	550
(15-min. mile, flat)	88	175	263	350
(20-min. mile, flat)	63	125	188	250
(20-min. mile, 4% incline)	100	200	300	400
Water aerobics	59	118	177	236
Weight lifting (vigorous)	89	177	266	354
Yoga	59	118	177	236

Formal, Functional, and Fun Exercises

Think about cleaning your house. Fact is, if you clean your house vigorously—dusting with passion, vacuuming with diligence, washing floors enthusiastically—you're also burning about sixty calories in fifteen minutes. I'm sure you've never before thought of housecleaning as exercise, but the next time you dread it, just shift your mind-set and remember that in a few hours of vigorous cleaning you can burn 800 calories.

Do you like to shop? Then how about speed walking through the mall or on a great shopping street? You can window-shop before actually going in the stores. Depending on your pace, you could burn 200 to 600 calories in an hour without even thinking of it as exercise. Even in an art museum, you can burn some calories just by getting the lay of the exhibits before slowing down to enjoy them leisurely.

What I'm hoping to point out to you with these examples is that you don't have to think of exercise in traditional terms; you can change the context of exercise—that is, how you relate to it.

Consider that there are three kinds of exercise: formal, functional, fun.

- **Formal exercise** is the kind you usually associate with going to the gym for aerobics classes and weight lifting, but also includes jogging, speed walking, swimming laps, etc.
- **Functional exercise** comes in many forms: gardening, cleaning house, parking a little farther away from work, and walking to do your errands, etc. Functional means you'd have to do these activities anyway, but now you get to think of them as helpful to your health.
- **Fun exercise** includes those activities you actually like doing for recreation: tennis, dancing, mountain biking, softball, kicking

the soccer ball around with the kids, etc. In other words, anything that gets you to play.

Almost everybody feels comfortable doing one or more activities from those three groups. The point being that if, like Tina, you're not one who loves to go for a four-mile jog, you can still find something that burns calories and moves your limbs.

Even for me, on those days when I can't find even a minute for my usual workout, I'll take my kids to the park for some playtime and, instead of sitting there reading a magazine while they play, I'll get out there on the grass with them and throw or kick the ball around. The idea is to inject more activity into your life—and then, using the fun or functional activities as rungs, to progress up the ladder toward more formal workouts by finding something that floats your boat.

Because in truth, if fitness is your goal, at some point you'll need to mix in formal activities with whatever else you have going on. Fun and functional activities don't generally give you enough of a cardiovascular workout by themselves. But you know what? In my experience, working with countless people, getting to formal exercise after starting with fun or functional activities happens almost automatically.

I know a woman who used to love going for leisurely Sunday bike rides with her kids. On other days when she was alone, she gradually stepped up the pace, until she'd become a legitimate bike racer. Coupling that with a weight program a few days a week, she became lean and fit rather quickly. And because she started something she liked, she didn't feel bored or discouraged. While she still enjoys those leisurely Sunday bike rides with her kids, she's now fit enough to appreciate how much progress she's made.

It's critically important to abandon the all-or-nothing thinking that plagues too many people. They believe that if they don't subject themselves to a full-tilt workout, then they might as well not do anything at all. That's not the way it has to work. As it turns out, a moderate but consistent approach is the one you're more likely to stick with for the long haul.

Both the Centers for Disease Control and the American College of Sports Medicine agree that an accumulated thirty minutes of activity—it can even be mixed between fun, functional, and formal exercise—five or six days a week will substantially reduce your risk factors for several diseases. So you can put together ten minutes of vigorous housecleaning with a ten-minute walk to or from work and ten minutes on a bicycle or treadmill or ten minutes of playing ball with your kids.

Starting this way is less likely to make you think of exercise as something that's unattainable or only for conditioned athletes. And you certainly don't have to feel guilty about not making it to the gym. Your goal is to incorporate exercise into your life the way you've incorporated bathing and brushing your teeth. After all, isn't exercise also a form of personal hygiene?

WHEN WILL YOU SEE RESULTS?

How quickly you begin to look and feel differently is determined by many factors, including your physiology and your commitment. For most people, however, the first noticeable change will occur within two weeks, and perhaps even ten days. You'll notice yourself having more energy, feeling more vital and alert, less tired, in a better mood. That's a huge motivator, because when you believe that your program is making a difference, you're more likely to continue it.

And if you continue it until the next step, you'll begin to see dramatic changes in your body. That typically happens after about four good weeks of working out consistently. Your body will begin to assume a more pleasing, toned shape, which is of course more impetus toward continuing your program.

After about three months, the first wave of dramatic results tends to level off. It's called plateauing, and everyone who's ever gotten into a program has gone through it. What's the symptom? Basically, you'll notice your body shaping progress slowing down. Beware, when you reach this point you may get somewhat discouraged and frustrated, and even start slacking off. (This is why starting a new fitness regime is easier than maintaining it.) But maintain you must. And you can.

To overcome those feelings of frustration, understand that plateauing is normal. It means that your body has actually adapted to your new exercise regime. It's humming, the cardiovascular system is operating more efficiently, with greater capacity. Your muscles have strengthened. If you stop now you'll lose that and basically have to start over.

My six-week plan will take you week by week through a fitness program that won't allow your body to settle into a routine that leads to plateauing. The variety built into the program not only keeps you motivated, but it's intended to keep you progressing week after week, so you can attain your fitness and weight goals and maintain them in the most efficient manner. My plan helps you avoid the slumps that throw you off target.

WHAT'S IN THE POWER OF CHOICE FITNESS PLAN?

It's time to put together your personal fitness plan consisting of three exercise categories:

- cardiovascular or aerobic
- strength training
- stretching and relaxation

To understand why any good fitness program has to include all three components, it helps to know why each one is important.

Cardiovascular or Aerobic Exercise

Cardiovascular or aerobic exercise is any type of rhythmic, continuous movement that uses the body's larger muscle groups (the legs and arms) for a sustained period—at least ten minutes, and up to an hour. By "rhythmic" I don't necessarily mean that it has to be done to music, though certainly aerobics classes are generally accompanied by music that has a driving beat because it motivates and inspires the exerciser the same way it does a dancer. Rhythmic in this case means that the activity—say, cycling or walking—is repeated, thus using the same muscle patterns over and over and over for the duration of the exercise.

The most important goal of cardiovascular or aerobic training is to condition the heart—that is, make it stronger and more efficient. Like the biceps or any other muscle in the body, the heart needs exercise to get stronger. You make it stronger by using the big muscle groups to raise your heart rate, which gets larger volumes of blood pumping back to the heart, keeping it conditioned. You know the old saying, "Use it or lose it"? Well, it applies to the heart as well. A less efficient heart can't deliver blood and oxygen to your muscles and brain as easily as a conditioned heart. Which is why a lack of regular aerobic training can badly hinder the cardiovascular system, or at least keep it from operating efficiently.

While heart conditioning is probably the most important benefit of aerobic exercise, the lungs, arteries, and veins also get stronger as oxygen is delivered in greater volume to every part of your body. And as they all get stronger, they, too, get more efficient, so that you continue to reap the benefits even when you're not exercising.

And then, of course, there's calorie-burning—which most people beginning an exercise regime tend to focus on. Aerobic exercise helps you develop the ability to burn fat. So people who work out aerobically can actually metabolize fat more efficiently.

No matter how intense your aerobic exercise, you will burn calories and can eventually lose fat weight. Obviously, though, the more strenuous the exercise, and the longer you do it, the more calories you burn.

Here's how your body works: Your body is burning calories throughout the day, whether you're active or resting. Even while resting, you burn (metabolize) about 1.5 calories per minute in order to satisfy your energy needs. Each calorie burned comes from both fat and carbohydrates, about 60 percent fat and 40 percent carbohydrates. But resting is not a very effective way to get rid of excess fat. For that you need exercise. A combination of aerobic exercise and strength training will help you burn more calories and therefore more total fat.

The key to proper aerobic exercise is to find a comfortable level, one appropriate to your fitness level, that you can maintain. But when I say "comfortable," I don't mean making it so easy that you end up cheating yourself out of all the good aerobics can do, including burning fat. You do have to push yourself a little in order to see those benefits.

A WORD OF ADVICE ON BUYING CARDIOVASCULAR EXERCISE EQUIPMENT

A good piece of exercise equipment can be a great investment in your health. But it's important to chose one that fits your personality. From a calorie-burning standpoint, the magic isn't in the piece of equipment itself, it's how hard and for how long you use it. Whether it's a treadmill or stair-stepper, most pieces of cardiovascular equipment can give you great results. But since you have to use them in order to get the benefit, you have to find a piece of equipment that you'll like. Would you enjoy riding a bike, cross-country skiing, walking on a treadmill, or climbing stairs? Ask yourself, before you buy.

After you've made that determination, do a little investigation into the size of the equipment. It sounds silly, but you'd be surprised how many people buy a piece of equipment that doesn't fit into their home. Either that, or they prefer it to be out of sight when not in use even though it wasn't designed to fold up into the size space they've allotted for hiding it. And, of course, be sensitive to pricing.

If you can exercise for an hour a day, six days a week, that would be great. But most people can't. So as you'll see in the cardiovascular section of my fitness plan, you'll need to put in from ten to sixty minutes at least three days a week. The minimum amounts are adequate to improve your overall health and reduce your cardiovascular risk factors. But if your goal is to substantially increase your fitness level, or improve your stamina, or to burn fat and lose weight, you need to work out a little more often and longer.

Strength Training

Strength training works by overloading a particular muscle, or muscle group, causing it to fatigue, which initiates a physiological reaction that leads to greater strength, improved muscle tone, and better muscle endurance.

I enthusiastically recommend strength training to people of all ages. It leads to greater strength, improved muscle tone, and better muscle endurance, not to mention increased bone density, and fewer fractures from osteoporosis.

There are other obvious benefits to strength training—such as being able to perform your daily tasks with greater ease—and some that are not so obvious: Strong muscles help prevent joint and muscle injuries and improve posture. Also, a lot of lower-back problems are significantly improved—and injuries prevented—with stronger muscles. And let's not forget about how your self-esteem will probably rise as your physical image improves.

Another often overlooked aspect of strength training is weight loss. It works this way: Efficient, lean muscles demand more energy than fat does, so increasing your lean muscle mass will increase your metabolic rate, both during exercise and at rest; either way, you'll burn more calories. The stronger you get, the more energy your muscles require to function, the more fat you'll burn off. This is why some men can eat three times as much food as their wives and not put on weight: Their muscles are significantly bigger. That additional muscle mass increases their metabolism and burns those added calories.

Some women shy away from weight training because they mistakenly believe that they'll necessarily end up looking muscle-bound. But it's not necessarily true. In general, men's muscle size increases as they get stronger because of large amounts of testosterone, which men have twenty to thirty times more of than women do. So women can increase their muscle strength with beautifully toned muscles that won't thicken them, and still get all the wonderful metabolic fat-burning benefits that men get. Those small gains in muscle size that do occur help shape the body, giving it the smooth, curvy legs and arms you want. Talk about a win-win situation.

Flexibility Training

Flexibility training is probably one of the most ignored components of physical fitness and overall personal health. But if you're flexible, you can do almost anything better, from driving a car to working out, since every joint and muscle in the body has an intended range of motion.

Stretching regularly (and properly) keeps your muscles long and supple. Typically, as we get older our muscles start to tighten, especially in some common areas: the back of your legs, your lower back, and your shoulder area. As this occurs your range of motion becomes limited and you develop aches and pains that weren't there before. Even everyday activities can become difficult. A flexible body moves easily through its proper range of motion, and requires less energy than a stiff or tight body.

Many people find that they can prevent soreness by stretching regularly after workouts, and they also report getting injured less frequently because injuries often occur when we try to push tight muscles through big movements that they haven't been prepared for. Stretching relaxes the muscle.

It also relieves stress. And you may discover that it alleviates chronic pain, the kind caused by poor posture created by muscle imbalances and tightness. If you cannot carry your body properly—if you can't maintain good, strong, upright posture—because a muscle or joint isn't flexible enough, your body has to compensate somehow, putting too much pressure on other parts of the body. A likely result of that is chronic pain, even injuries. So by going to the source, stretching out those tight, inflexible joints and muscles, you can regain the kind of posture your parents tried to instill in you.

Stretching from just five to twenty minutes, two to four times a week, makes a huge difference in your flexibility. In my plan, I'll show you how to incorporate your stretching routine into your aerobic and strength-training workouts. How? At the end of a twenty-minute walking workout, for example, you could get in three or four stretches for the lower body muscles that you just worked hard during the routine. And while you're doing your strength workout, you can use your rest time between sets or exercises to stretch your body. Of course, if you want to focus on the relaxation and stress-reduction benefits of stretching, which is what I like to do, do your stretching in one continuous routine for which you've set aside time.

Designing Your Power of Choice Fitness Plan

Determining Your Workout Level

As it is with eating, having exercise choices is a key ingredient of a successful fitness program. I've created guidelines that give you the ability to choose from a variety of activities as a way of preventing boredom and keeping you motivated. For those of you who are more comfortable with a "prescription" for your fitness program, I've developed a unique walking plan called the Lean Walk System. Remember, even if you use my walking system, in time you'll want to include your own choices for activities to create excitement and variety.

My Power of Choice Fitness Plan is designed for all fitness levels, covers aerobic conditioning, strength training, and stretching, and it's divided into three categories:

- Just Starting Out
- Exercise a Little
- Exercise Regularly

"Just Starting Out" is for people who haven't exercised in the last year, or who are coming back after a break. This is also a good place to go when you need to temporarily scale back.

Those in the "Exercise a Little" category are more active, but aren't as consistent with their workouts.

"Exercise Regularly" people have already developed the discipline to stick with a program.

It's possible you might be an "Exercise Regularly" in aerobics, but "Just Starting Out" in strength training, or any combination of these categories.

To create your own personal fitness program, start by deciding which level is most appropriate for you, then look at each exercise category on the chart (aerobic, strength, stretching) to determine how frequently you're going to work out and how long you're going to work out.

I can't emphasize enough how important it is to be honest with yourself when beginning. Whether you're starting from scratch, or you already exercise a little, or you exercise regularly and want a greater challenge, you have to choose the category most appropriate for you. Please believe me, you don't get any extra points for putting yourself in a higher level than you should be in. And you could set yourself up for discouragement, and possibly injury. If you're in doubt, err on the side of caution. **As always, check with your doctor before beginning any exercise program.**

THE POWER OF CHOICE WORKOUT SCHEDULE

	JUST STARTING OUT	EXERCISE A LITTLE	EXERCISE REGULARLY
Aerobic (Page 199)			
Frequency	2–3 times/week	3–4 times/week	4–6 times/week
Duration	10–20 minutes	20–30 minutes	30–60 minutes
Activity	1 activity	1 or 2 activities	1–3 activities
	or	or	or
	Lean Walk System	Lean Walk System	Lean Walk System

(Remember, in the aerobics category you can choose any aerobic activity or follow my Lean Walk System.)

	JUST STARTING OUT	EXERCISE A LITTLE	EXERCISE REGULARLY
Strength (Page 226)			
Frequency	2–3 days/week	3 days/week	4 days/week
Duration	10–15 minutes	15–20 minutes	20–30 minutes
Activity	7–9 exercises	10–15 exercises	15–20 exercises
	1 set/exercise	1 set/exercise	1–2 sets/exercise
Stretching (Page 268)			
Frequency	2 days/week	3 days/week	4 days/week
Duration	5–10 minutes	5–15 minutes	5–20 minutes
Activity	5 stretches	5–6 stretches	5–8 stretches

So let's get started setting up your own personal fitness plan, one designed around your needs and tastes. Your plan will include aerobic, strength, and stretching each week. First, I want you to be comfortable determining your workout schedule, so let's take a look at a hypothetical situation, using one of my friends, Kate.

FITNESS PLAN EXAMPLE

Kate has been away from exercise for several months, so she is "Just Starting Out." She begins by referring to the column with the "Just Starting Out" heading. First, she sees that she will be doing aerobics, two to three times a week, for ten to twenty minutes per session. She can choose one of the aerobic activities listed on page 199 (refer to aerobic activity chart), or use my Lean Walk System, on page 213.

Next, for strength training, she'll be working out two to three days a week, and doing from seven to nine exercises. She has the option of doing her aerobic and strength training on the same day, or doing her aerobics one day, and strength training the next.

Finally, Kate will be stretching two days a week, doing five stretches per workout. She can do these stretches after her aerobic and strength-training workouts, or might prefer to spend a little more time and stretch on her off days. As a mom with three kids, one of the benefits of the program for Kate is that it provides her the flexibility to plan workouts around her schedule.

WARMING UP

You've probably heard for years that warming up before exercising is essential, but you may not have understood why.

Warming up prepares your body for the activity ahead. By gradually raising your heart rate and increasing your body temperature, it actually makes the workout more efficient. Starting out too fast can cause lactic acid—that burning feeling in your muscles—to occur, and could interfere with your overall workout because you need to recover.

During your warm-up, more blood travels to the working muscles, which prepares your body for the workout ahead. That's why warming up makes the exercise more efficient. What's more, warm muscles stretch easier, so you're less likely to injure or strain them as you exercise.

To warm up properly, choose an easy, rhythmic activity for at least five minutes before the workout. Probably the easiest warm-up is to do the same activity you're going to be doing during the workout, but at a slower, easier pace. So if, for instance, you plan to walk briskly for thirty minutes, start out walking more slowly for five minutes, then gradually gain speed.

If you find that you like to stretch a bit during your warm-up, be sure you do so gently. Avoid sudden movements because your muscles and tendons aren't ready yet. Really, the best time to stretch is *after* your workout, when your muscles are warm and ready to lengthen.

THE LEAN WALK SYSTEM

My Lean Walk System is a complete aerobic program designed around one of my favorite activities—walking. It's a true "no-excuse workout." Lean Walk consists of three progressive walking workouts: Lean Walk I, Lean Walk II, and Lean Walk III. It also incorporates a dynamic concept in exercise called periodization.

PERIODIZATION

Periodization is a proven, scientific method of training that elite athletes use in order to "peak" just before big events.

In simple terms, periodization is a valuable tool that can help you get the most out of your exercise program, especially if you've hit a "plateau"— the place where, though you continue to work out, you stop seeing progress. It works by varying one or more of the three key aspects of your workout—length, activity, and intensity. By changing what you ask your body to do, periodization challenges you so you keep making fitness progress. Think of periodization as your personal training secret. You can apply the first two concepts of periodization (length and intensity) to most aerobic activities by simply adapting the following walking guidelines to the activity of your choice.

Changing the aerobic activity itself is also a form of periodization, now popularly called cross-training. It, too, can lift you off a plateau.

Let's get started with the Lean Walk System using walking as the aerobic activity. Each week we'll be adjusting either the duration or intensity of our workouts. I've used this technique over the years when I want to increase my fitness level, break the monotony of doing the same routine, and get off a plateau. Remember, you can use this periodization plan with any aerobic activity.

WEEK 1

Begin with Lean Walk I.

LEAN WALK I

This walking level is designed to get you off the couch and onto your feet. It will build stamina and endurance, as well as provide a good base from which you can progress to the next two walking programs.

Walk I gets you going at a comfortable, steady pace, at which you can carry on a conversation. Depending on your level of fitness ("Just Starting Out," "Exercise a Little," "Exercise Regularly"), you'll be walking anywhere from ten to sixty minutes at a pace that meets your fitness level. If you have the time and are a more experienced exerciser, go longer.

Before you start the program, determine the time it takes you to walk one mile so that you have a baseline against which to measure progress. At the beginning, at least, don't worry how fast you go or how long it takes. Find a comfortable route, mark off a mile, and record the time. Lean Walk I starts off with an easy five-minute warm-up, comparable to a strolling pace. Then try to increase your pace slightly so you're walking faster than your "strolling" pace. This is your "steady-state" pace. Monitor your intensity using the Rating of Perceived Exertion chart on page 222. Stay close to the 4–5 level.

LEAN WALK I

5 min.	10–50 minutes	5 min.
Warm-Up Pace	Steady-State Pace	Cool-Down Pace

(Steady-State Pace intensity will change as you progress)

During Lean Walk I, you're building your foundation. To do that you have to develop good walking techniques. Here are the essentials.

- **Posture.** Stand tall, imagine a string coming from the top of your head pulling you up. Then tilt your body forward slightly from the ankles, not the hips or waist. Don't arch your lower back or stick your butt out. Keep your spine in a neutral position by contracting your abdominals.
- **Head Position.** Don't tilt your head from side to side, and don't drop your chin forward. Your eyes should focus straight ahead and not on your feet, so you don't strain your neck.
- **Shoulders.** Your shoulders should be down and back; open your chest for easier, deeper breathing. As you walk, check your shoulders regularly. Are you slouching? Are your shoulders creeping up toward your ears?
- **Arms.** Let your arms swing freely, but with purpose. It improves your balance, increases circulation, and burns more calories. Swing your arms forward, not across your body. Imagine your body on a clock face, viewed from the side, with your head at twelve o'clock. Your arms should swing from seven o'clock (just behind your hips) to four o'clock (about belly button height).
- **Feet.** Strike the ground with your heel and let your foot roll forward naturally. At the end of your stride, really push off with your toes, to propel your body forward. Use a stride length that's comfortable for you. Don't overstride.

Focus on walking at a moderate, steady-state pace, using proper form and technique. If you feel that you want to do more, go ahead and increase your walk by five to ten minutes, keeping the intensity moderate.

If you're working out "aerobically" more than four times a week, feel free to choose another activity for one or two workouts, just to get some variety going. **Before moving on to Lean Walk II, you should be able to complete a mile in twenty minutes or less.**

Continue with Lean Walk I and keep increasing your speed until you reach this goal. For it to be effective, you have to have established a good, firm base of fitness, which you can do only when you exercise regularly.

WEEK 2

Continue with Lean Walk I, but lengthen your walks by ten to twenty minutes. Your focus this week is on building your endurance through longer training. Maintain a comfortable pace.

WEEK 3

Now it's time to move on to Lean Walk II.

WALK II

This level is a step up. It will increase your endurance and fitness, and burn a greater number of calories than you burned in Lean Walk I. You'll be walking faster, too, completing a mile in no more than 15 to 17 minutes.

Unless you're sure that you're in pretty good shape, stay in Lean Walk I for a few weeks before trying out Lean Walk II, because this program uses "aerobic intervals" as a way of pushing you to work a little harder for short amounts of time within your twenty to thirty minute workout.

Here's how it works: Warm up for five to ten minutes. Begin your warm-up and build to your steady-state pace during that time. Then it's time to start the interval workouts.

Speed up until you feel you're working just a bit harder than would otherwise be comfortable. This is considered your AEROBIC INTERVAL. You should be pushing between 6–7 on the Rating of Perceived Exertion chart on page 222.

Maintain this aerobic interval for three minutes. Then return to your steady-state pace for three minutes. This is called your RECOVERY INTERVAL.

Continue these interval cycles—three minutes of aerobic interval pace (pushing yourself slightly), followed by three minutes of recovery—for twenty to twenty-four minutes. You should be able to complete from two to four cycles of intervals.

Then finish your walk at an easy pace in order to cool down.

LEAN WALK II

5–10 min.	3 min.	3 min.	3 min.	3 min.	5–10 min.
Warm-Up Pace	Aerobic Interval	**Recovery Interval**	Aerobic Interval	**Recovery Interval**	Cool-Down Pace

(To increase intensity and duration, add one to two additional
aerobic intervals)

As you get fitter and fitter, you can choose to work harder by walking faster during the aerobic intervals. Just make sure, though, that you slow down to a moderate level during the recovery intervals.

If at the end of a three-minute work interval you think you could have gone longer, then you're ready to walk a little faster. The key is, you should be ready to recover at the end of each work interval.

In Lean Walk II, you also need to adjust your technique to reflect your greater speed. Make your movements more efficient, and the workout itself more beneficial. Here are some tips to help increase your speed.

- **Arm Swing.** Since your arms and legs work in unison, your legs can't speed up until your arms do. To get your arms pumping more quickly, start by putting a 90-degree bend in your elbow, holding your hands in a loose fist. Swing forward, not side to side, keeping elbows close to your side.
- **Feet.** Use the same rolling heel-toe motion as in Walk I, but concentrate on actively pulling up your toes as your legs swing forward. At faster paces, if you don't pull up your toes, you'll start catching them on the ground.

Remember to walk fast enough during each aerobic interval so that it feels like a pretty hard workout—but not so fast that you can't complete the three minutes. To find just the right pace, a lot of people end up experimenting. Don't worry. You'll end up at your proper speed.

For the recovery intervals, return to your comfortable, steady-state pace. But try not to slow down as much as you would during the cool down at the end of your walk.

What I love about this phase is that you start out at a comfortable pace, one that doesn't leave you breathless. But as you start your aerobic interval, you have to focus for those three minutes in order to push yourself faster than you'd normally go. It takes concentration—and probably some perspiration. You'll feel out of breath, and at the end of the three minutes be ready to slow down for your recovery intervals.

WEEK 4

Stick with Walk II. But if you can, increase your walks by ten to twenty minutes. What that gives you is one to two more aerobic intervals cycles, so you'll be challenging both your intensity and duration levels.

If you can't increase intensity and duration, just lengthen your walk—and while you're completing the added distance, proceed at your steady-state pace.

WEEK 5

You've now graduated to Lean Walk III.

WALK III

This level is designed as an advanced program to increase your aerobic fitness level as you go faster. And, of course, it burns a ton of calories.

Before beginning Lean Walk III, make sure you've spent enough time in the first two phases so that you've built enough endurance and practiced your techniques. This is necessary because Lean Walk III is a reasonably strenuous program, for even the fittest people. Lean Walk III uses ANAEROBIC INTERVALS to challenge you. Anaerobic intervals are short, intense exercise periods that really push you to the next level of fitness.

> The word AEROBIC means "with oxygen." Aerobic exercises are those that use continuous motion for an extended period of time, such as jogging, cycling, walking, etc.
>
> The word ANAEROBIC means "without sufficient oxygen." Anaerobic exercises are more intense but of shorter duration. They quickly push you past your aerobic threshold, leaving you breathless. Some examples are weight training, sprinting, or short but intense periods of typical aerobic activities.

Begin your Lean Walk III with a five- to ten-minute warm-up, building to a steady-state pace. Then do two cycles of AEROBIC INTERVALS from Lean Walk II—three minutes of pushing slightly more than your steady-state, followed by three minutes of recovery (at a moderate level).

Now you're ready for an ANAEROBIC INTERVAL: Walk as fast as you possibly can for one minute. On your perceived exertion scale, you'll get up to the 7–9 level during the fast part of the interval. Then drop down to a brisk, moderate pace for the three-minute RECOVERY INTERVAL.

By design, the one-minute anaerobic interval should push you to your maximum effort. No holding back!

The three-minute recovery allows you to catch your breath a bit . . . and get ready for your next interval.

Make it a goal to do three to five cycles of these anaerobic intervals. Finish with a cool down at a steady pace for the remainder of your workout time.

LEAN WALK III

5–10 min.	3 min.	3 min.	3 min.	3 min.	1 min.	3 min.	1 min.	3 min.	1 min.	3 min.	5–10 min.
Warm-Up Pace	Aerobic Interval	Recovery Interval	Aerobic Interval	Recovery Interval	Anaerobic Interval	Recovery Interval	Anaerobic Interval	Recovery Interval	Anaerobic Interval	Recovery Interval	Cool-Down Pace

(To increase the intensity and duration, add one or two additional anaerobic intervals)

When you feel comfortable with this program, alternate aerobic and anaerobic intervals for the duration of your walk. But always remember to begin and end your workout at a nice, steady pace.

If, during the anaerobic intervals, you feel awkward or less than coordinated, you may have to adjust your technique slightly. Here are a few tips.

- **Arms.** Keep your arms close to your side and start pumping them more quickly. As you start to go faster, your arms will swing across your body slightly, and that's okay.
- **Walk the Line.** Up until now, you've been walking with your feet parallel. To increase your speed, try to make your feet land, one in front of the other, so you're walking a straight line. If you were walking on an actual line, just the inside of your foot (the instep) would touch the line.
- **Hips.** "Walking the line" forces you to rotate your pelvis, and extend your hips slightly, which lengthens your stride a little. Just align your footsteps, leading with your heels, and stay loose in your pelvis as your hips follow where your legs lead.

I wouldn't be at all surprised if you could do only one or two of these all-out intervals. So progress cautiously and slowly, adding interval cycles as you feel you can.

If you're going to work out five or six days this week, alternate one day of Lean Walk III with a day of Lean Walk I.

WEEK 6

Stick with Lean Walk III for this, the last week of your high-intensity training phase. No doubt you'll feel ready to recover next week.

This week, keep your duration as it was in Week 5, but try to fit one or two more anaerobic intervals into your workout. That means you should do a little bit less steady-state walking between intervals; your goal is to keep them closer together.

As in Week 5, alternate high-intensity days with moderate-levels days, or else change activities on the alternate days.

NOW WHAT?

Congratulations!

You've completed an entire six-week cycle and are now ready to start a new one. Go back to Week 1 and bring your focus from hard to moderate. And again, you'll increase the length of your workouts as you feel ready. Remember that this six-week cycle works not only for walking but also for any aerobic activity. Try it with cycling, running, and stepping, to name just a few activities.

I highly recommend taking at least a couple of days this week to go easily. Just cruise at a comfortable pace and enjoy the scenery as you marvel at how much easier it is for you now than it was six weeks ago. You might want to invite a friend along.

PLATEAUS

From beginner to elite, everyone hits a plateau now and then. On that plateau, you feel that you're not making any progress, and that you'll never again make progress because you've gone as far as you can go; this is it, this is the limit of your potential. You're stuck, destined, it seems, to remain here forever. You're not getting any fitter, and maybe your weight loss has slowed as well.

Well, guess what?

The reason your body plateaus is that it has become more efficient, more capable of handling the same routine; it doesn't have to work as hard to get the workout done. Since it's not being challenged, it stays at the same level.

So what can you do to get back to the kind of progress that felt so good and was so motivating? Periodization. Your six-week Lean Walk System is designed to keep you off those plateaus, and the variety will keep you motivated.

RATING OF PERCEIVED EXERTION

Rating of Perceived Exertion is a way to estimate how hard you're working by simply taking stock of how you're feeling—changes in breathing, heart rate, sweating, and fatigue—and then rating those sensations on a scale from one ("very, very light") to ten ("very, very hard"). The advantage of this over taking your pulse is that you don't have to stop exercising to measure your exertion.

To rate your perceived exertion, just think about how you feel as you're walking: Do your legs feel like they're hardly working, or do they hurt? Are you breathing hard? Is your heart pounding? Are you sweating? Then assign a number to your observation, as follows:

No.	Amount of Exertion
1–2	Very, very light
3	Very light
4	Moderate
5	Somewhat hard
6	Hard
7–8	Very hard
9–10	Very, very hard

During your walks try to stay in the 1–6 range unless otherwise directed. (Beginning exercisers should be closer to 4.) Warm-up and cool down should be between 2 and 3.

STRENGTH-TRAINING EXERCISES

It takes only ten to thirty minutes of strength workouts, two to four days per week, to see great results. That means doing anywhere from seven to twenty exercises every workout. Choosing one exercise for each of the major muscle groups in your body, and doing one set of each exercise, is all you have to do. That small time and effort commitment pays such great dividends.

Remember, though, that your muscles need forty-eight hours to recover from a strength-training workout. So don't work out two days in a row—unless you're working out different muscles, say, upper body one day, lower body the next.

You may be wondering how to fit your strength workouts together with your aerobic workouts. The answer depends on your individual schedule. Some people prefer doing their cardiovascular workout first, so that their muscles are warm and ready for their strength training. Others like to alternate aerobic days with strength-training days. Time, or lack of it, is probably the critical factor here.

HOW MANY REPETITIONS AND HOW MUCH WEIGHT?

Figuring out how many repetitions (or "reps," as they're known in the gym) you have to perform on each exercise takes a bit of trial and error. A good, safe guideline to follow is to choose a weight that allows you to complete between twelve and twenty repetitions—until the muscle being worked feels almost completely fatigued. You've completed a good set when the muscle starts to feel tired but you can still maintain good form and technique on every repetition. If your technique becomes sloppy, you either began with too much weight or performed too many repetitions. Adding more repetitions with bad technique won't make you stronger. It may, however, cause injury.

An exercise's intensity is relative to your current strength level, so you may start out with the easiest variations of an exercise, or with a lighter weight, and feel fatigued in ten to twelve repetitions. That will be perfect to start with. Because as you get stronger—and you will, quickly—you'll find that you're no longer fatigued at ten to twelve repetitions (one set) . . . so you'll have to increase the exercise's intensity. You do that by adding weight or changing the body position. Then go back to your ten to twelve repetitions. You should feel fatigued, but this time you're a step higher on the strength ladder, and continuing to climb.

We're going to start you with only one set of each exercise, though as you progress and get stronger, you may want at some point to do two sets of each. This extended workout obviously takes more time, but it will give you additional strength results as well as better calorie-burning.

A word of caution, though. While I encourage you to build over time to two sets, please understand that, no matter how fit you're getting, moving to three or more sets actually has diminishing results. Two sets of each exercise may be twice as good as one set, but three sets is absolutely not three times better. Yes, experienced body builders or other elite athletes with specific training goals may do more than two sets, but their programs have been designed with their individual performance goals in mind.

Take a look at the following chart to get a better idea of what is expected of a beginning, intermediate, and advanced program:

STRENGTH-TRAINING REPETITION GUIDELINES

Just starting out	Exercising a little	Exercising regularly
12 to 20 reps to mild fatigue	10 to 15 reps to moderate fatigue	8 to 12 reps to moderate fatigue

The following exercises are listed in the order that you'll be performing them.

If you're a beginner, choose just the first seven to nine exercises. Then, as you progress, continue to add exercises (in the order listed).

Please note that several of these exercises require the use of dumbbells. What you buy depends on your strength level. If you've never lifted weights before, you might start with three-pound dumbbells, eventually moving up to five pounds. Don't be afraid of buying heavier dumbbells, because once you start and lift regularly, you'll be using ten- and even fifteen-pound dumbbells. Throughout the following exercise descriptions, I'll show you the starting position, tell you how to perform the exercise with proper technique, and show you how to make the exercise more difficult when you are ready to progress.

STRENGTH EXERCISES

1. Push-up

Works your chest, front of shoulders, and back of upper arm.

Starting Position: Kneel on the ground with your arms lined up so that your wrists are directly beneath your shoulders and fingertips turned in slightly. Walk your hands forward until your body is at an angle from your knees up to your shoulders. Keep your neck straight.

The Exercise: Inhale, and bend your elbows, lowering your body down until your chest nears the floor. Pause, exhale, and press back up to starting position.

Technique Tips: Hold your abdominal muscles in tight so that your body is in a straight line as you lower it. Don't let your back sag as your arms get tired. Keep your shoulders over your wrists the whole time; avoid the tendency to push your weight back when you get tired. If you can't lower your body all the way down, start with a quarter push-up and gradually progress lower.

How to Make It Harder: When the kneeling push-up gets easy, straighten out your legs and balance on your toes.

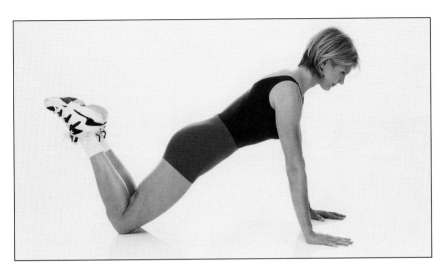

Push-up Position A

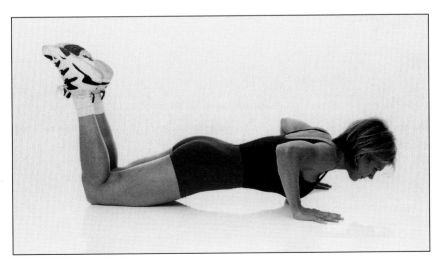

Push-up Position B

2. One-Arm Row

Works your middle back, upper back, rear of shoulder, and front of upper arm.

Starting Position: Use your medium dumbbell. Stand with your feet in a staggered position on the floor with your left foot forward. Lean forward and place your left hand on the seat of a chair in front of your left knee. Keep your back straight and parallel to the floor. Your right arm should hang straight down, dumbbell in hand.

The Exercise: Exhale, and bend your elbow, lifting the dumbbell until your elbow is higher than your back and the dumbbell is close to your underarm. Keep your palm facing your body. Pause at the top, inhale, and lower back down.

Technique Tips: Keep your palm facing in and your elbow pointing back—don't let it swing out to the side. Also, keep both shoulders facing the floor; don't let your body tip to the side.

How to Make It Harder: Use your heavier dumbbell and complete the exercise with the same technique.

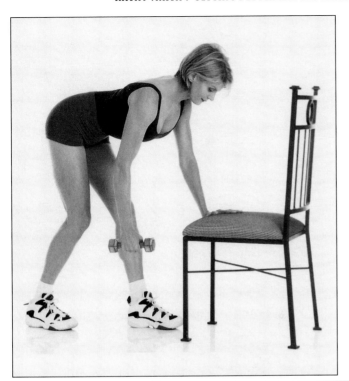

*One-Arm Row
Position A*

*One-Arm Row
Position B*

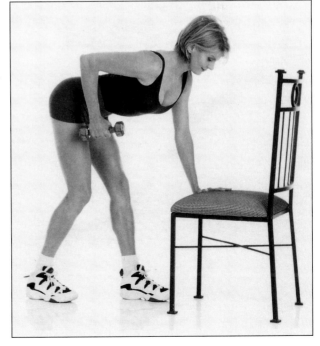

3. Back Extension

Works your lower back muscles.

Starting Position: Lie on your stomach with your feet down and forehead resting on your hands, elbows out to the side.

The Exercise: Keeping your neck straight, exhale, and slowly lift your chest off the floor using your lower back muscles. Pause at the top, inhale, and lower back to starting position.

Technique Tips: Keep the tops of your feet on floor—don't kick your legs up into a "Superman" position! That can place excess stress on your lower back. Don't lift your head; concentrate on using those back muscles to raise your torso. Keep your eyes focused on the floor and your elbows out to the side. Lift only as high as you comfortably can—an inch or two is fine.

How to Make It Harder: Extend your arms up over your head and clasp your hands together. As you lift your chest off the floor, squeeze your upper arms in close to your ears.

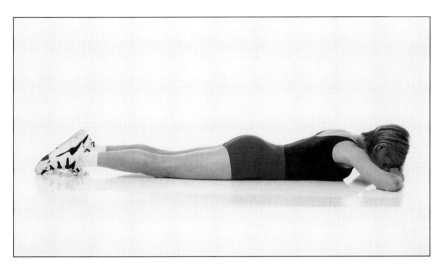

Back Extension Position A

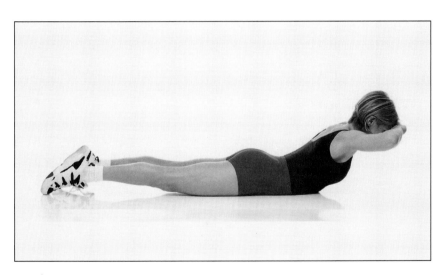

Back Extension Position B

4. Crunch

Works your abdominal muscles.

Starting Position: Lie on your back with your knees bent and feet flat on the floor. Place your hands behind your head, and keep your neck relaxed; don't push your chin up or pull it down into your chest. Keep your elbows comfortably out to the side.

The Exercise: Exhale, tighten your abdominals, and pull your rib cage down toward your hips, lifting your head, neck, and shoulder blades off the ground as one unit. Remember: This isn't an old-fashioned sit-up—you don't need to lift more than a few inches off the floor. Pause at the top of the movement, then inhale as you slowly lower all the way back down.

Technique Tips: Concentrate on pulling your rib cage down, as opposed to lifting your head and shoulders up. Make sure the movement comes from your abs—not your neck or shoulders. Use your hands only to *support* your head, not lift it.

How to Make It Harder: Extend your arms overhead and clasp your hands together. As you crunch, squeeze your upper arms in close to your ears.

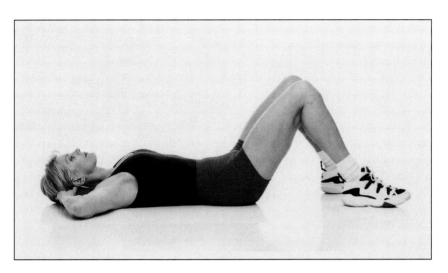

Crunch Position A

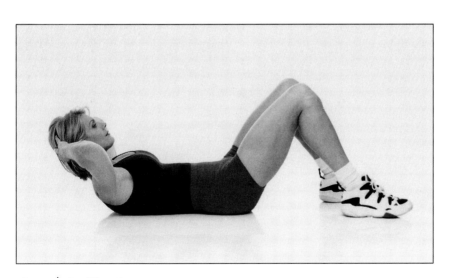

Crunch Position B

5. Cross Crunch

Works your waist and abdominal muscles.

Starting Position: Lie on your back with your knees bent and feet flat on the floor. Place your hands behind your head, elbows comfortably out to the side, and keep your neck relaxed, as in the Crunch.

The Exercise: Exhale. As you curl your head, neck, and shoulder blades off the floor, rotate your torso, pulling the left side of your rib cage toward your right inner thigh. Pause at the top, inhale, and slowly lower back down. Repeat, alternating sides. Be sure to do the recommended number of repetitions *for each side*.

Technique Tips: Make sure you rotate only your torso—not your arms and neck. Keep your elbows in line with your ears throughout the movement. Concentrate on pulling your rib cage down and across rather than pulling your elbows across.

How to Make It Harder: Do all the repetitions on one side, then repeat the same number on the other side. Do not alternate sides between each repetition.

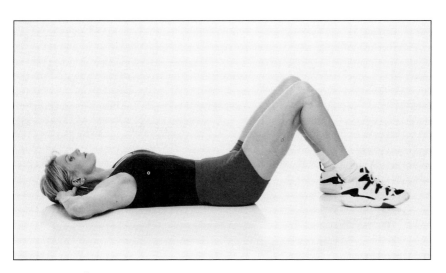

Cross Crunch Position A

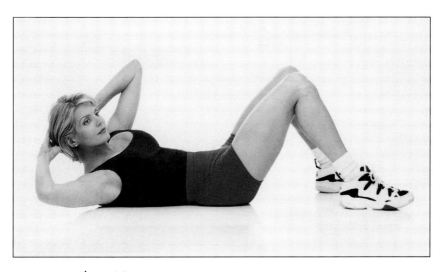

Cross Crunch Position B

6. Squat

Works the front and rear thigh muscles and buttocks.

Starting Position: Stand up straight with your abdominals tightened, feet hip-width apart and hands by your sides.

The Exercise: Inhale, bend your knees as if you're going to sit in a chair, and lower down until your thighs are nearly parallel to the floor. Meanwhile, lift your arms out in front of you for balance. Pause, exhale, and slowly stand up.

Technique Tips: As you lower down, make sure your tailbone points back. Keep your chest lifted and back straight, not rounded. Finally, don't let your knees shoot out past your toes.

How to Make It Harder: Use your medium to heavy dumbbells. Hold them by your sides as you squat, rather than reaching out in front of you.

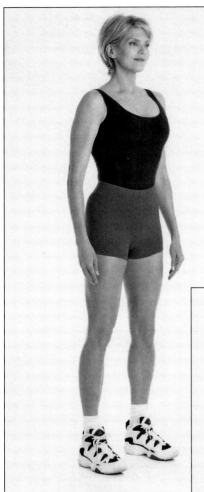

Squat Position A

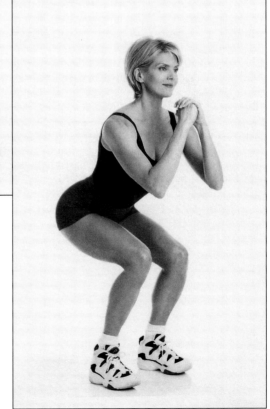

Squat Position B

7. Hamstring Curl

Works rear thigh muscles and buttocks.

Starting Position: Lie on your back with your knees bent and heels on the seat of a chair. Your lower legs should be parallel to the ground, thighs perpendicular. Place your arms on the floor for balance.

The Exercise: Exhale, and press your heels down into the chair as if you were pulling them toward the back of your thighs. Keep pushing them down until your hips lift off the floor. Pause at the top, inhale, and slowly lower back down.

Technique Tips: Make your hamstrings do the work. Rather than using your buttocks to push your hips, really squeeze your heels down.

How to Make It Harder: Hold your medium to heavy dumbbells in your hands and rest them on the front of your hips, right where your hips bend.

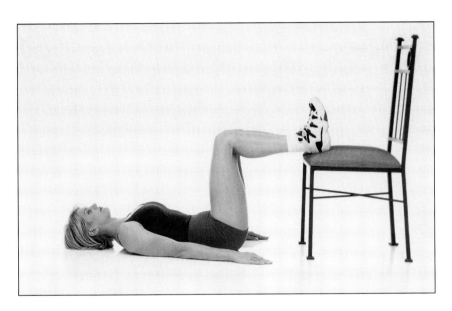

Hamstring Curl Position A

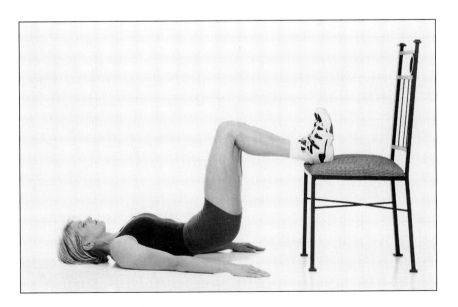

Hamstring Curl Position B

8. Seated Biceps Curl

Works the front of your upper arm.

Starting Position: Use your medium dumbbells. Sit up straight in a chair with your feet flat on the floor. Hold a dumbbell in each hand with your arms hanging by your sides, palms facing in.

The Exercise: Exhale, and slowly bend your elbows, curling the dumbbells up to your shoulders. As you bend your elbows, gradually rotate your palms so that at the top of the movement they are facing your shoulders. Inhale, and slowly lower back down.

Technique Tips: As you curl the dumbbells, keep your elbows close to your sides. Don't swing your arms back and forth from the shoulder.

How to Make It Harder: Use your heavier dumbbells.

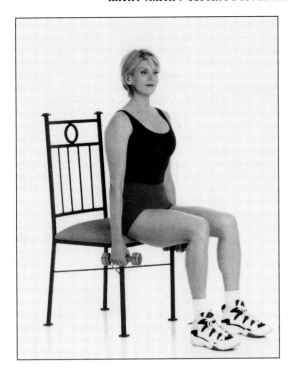

Seated Biceps Curl
Position A

Seated Biceps Curl
Position B

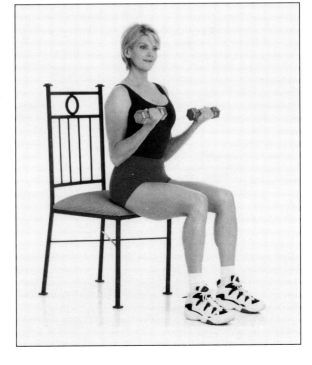

9. Triceps Kickback

Works the back of your upper arm.

Starting Position: Use your light to medium dumbbells. Lean forward, place your left hand on the seat of a chair, and stagger your feet so your left leg is in front of your right and both knees are slightly bent. Holding a dumbbell in your right hand, lift your arm until your elbow is slightly higher than your body and the dumbbell points to the floor, palm facing in.

The Exercise: Exhale, then slowly straighten your elbow until your arm is straight. Pause at the top of the movement, inhale, and return to starting position.

Technique Tips: Throughout the exercise, keep your upper arm still, your back straight, and both shoulders facing the floor.

How to Make It Harder: Use your medium to heavy dumbbell.

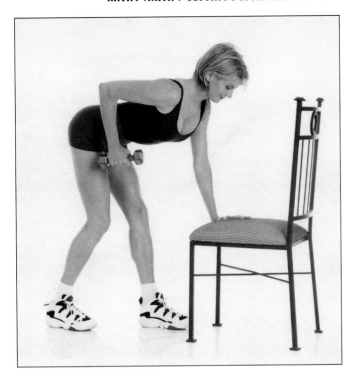

*Triceps
Kickback
Position A*

*Triceps
Kickback
Position B*

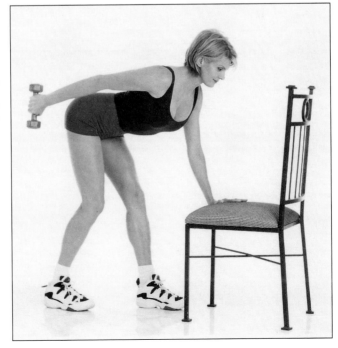

10. Lateral Raise

Works the center shoulder muscles.

Starting Position: Use your light or medium dumbbells. Stand with your feet hip-width apart, knees slightly bent, abdominals tightened, and arms hanging by your sides. Hold a dumbbell in each hand, palms facing in.

The Exercise: Exhale, and slowly lift your arms out to the side until your elbows are even with your shoulders. Pause, inhale, and slowly lower back down.

Technique Tips: Lift directly out to the side; don't let the dumbbells end up in front of your thighs. At the top of the movement, let your thumbs turn slightly upward. Keep your elbows slightly bent, not locked.

How to Make It Harder: Use your medium to heavy dumbbells.

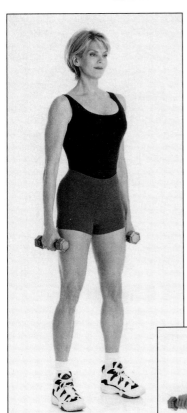

Lateral Raise
Position A

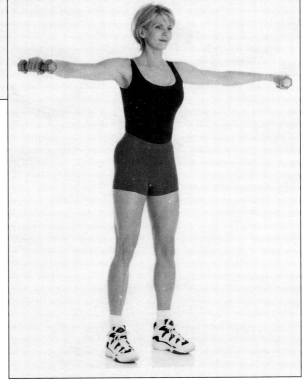

Lateral Raise
Position B

11. Inner Thigh Pull

Works your inner thigh muscles.

Starting Position: Stand with your feet wide enough apart to feel a slight stretch in your inner thighs. Bend your knees, turn your toes out slightly, tighten your abdominals, and place your hands on your hips.

The Exercise: Exhale, and drag your right foot toward your left foot, using the floor as resistance. Keep dragging until your feet are together and legs are straight, with your toes turned out slightly (like "first position" in ballet). Inhale, take a wide step to the side with your *left* foot, then drag it in. Continue alternating legs.

Technique Tips: Drag your foot enough so that you really feel your inner thigh muscles working. Imagine that you have one foot on a dock and the other foot on a boat three feet away, and you're trying to pull the boat into the dock. Keep the sole of your foot flat on the floor; don't drag the inside of your shoe.

How to Make It Harder: Step out into a slightly wider position and bend your knees a little deeper as you start. "Drag" with the same amount of resistance described above.

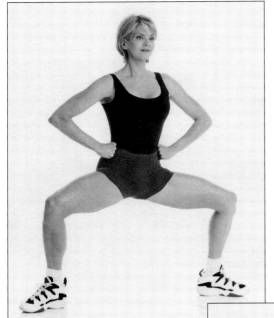

*Inner Thigh Pull
Position A*

*Inner Thigh Pull
Position B*

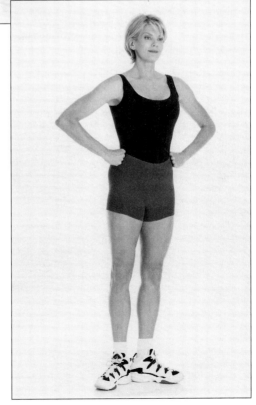

12. Standing Side Lift

Works your outer hip muscles.

Starting Position: Stand up straight with your abdominals tight-ened and your left side facing the back of a chair. Lean slightly to the side, resting your left elbow on the chair. Bring your right arm across your body, placing your hand on the top of the chair for bal-ance.

The Exercise: Exhale, and slowly lift your right leg out to the side, keeping your knee and foot facing forward. Lift as high as you can without turning your knee and toe up to the ceiling. Pause at the top, inhale, and lower back down.

Technique Tips: Make sure your leg is lifting directly out to the side, not behind you. Your supporting leg muscles are working to keep you balanced and upright.

How to Make It Harder: Attach medium to heavy ankle weights just above the knee or at the ankle.

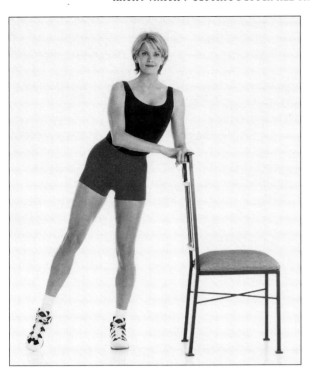

*Standing
Side Lift
Position A*

*Standing
Side Lift
Position B*

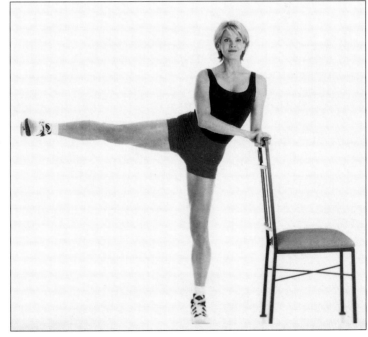

13. Reverse Curl

Works the lower region of your abdominal muscles.

Starting Position: Lie on your back with your knees lined up directly over hips. Your heels should hang down near the back of your thighs. Rest your arms on the floor beside you at your side, palms facing down.

The Exercise: Exhale, tighten your abdominals, and tilt your hips off the floor. Pause at the top of the move, inhale, and lower back down. This is a subtle move—your hips barely need to clear the floor.

Technique Tips: Concentrate on lifting with the lower part of your abdominal muscles, *not* your front hip muscles. Don't kick or swing your legs. Try not to push on the floor with your hands.

How to Make It Harder: Clasp your hands behind your head and lift your upper body off the floor in a crunch as you simultaneously perform the reverse curl.

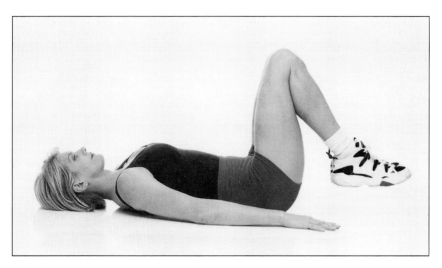

Reverse Curl Position A

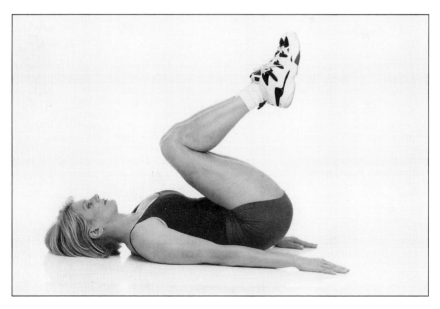

Reverse Curl Position B

14. Seated Back Flye

Works the upper back and rear of shoulders.

Starting Position: Use your light dumbbells. Sit on a chair with a pillow on your lap and lean forward, letting your chest rest on the pillow. Grasping your dumbbells, let your arms hang down to the sides. (Practice this exercise a few times with no dumbbells.)

The Exercise: Exhale, squeeze your shoulder blades together, and slowly lift your arms out to the side until they're slightly higher than shoulder level. Pause, inhale, and lower back down.

Technique Tips: Make sure your arms lift directly out to the side, not behind you. Keep your shoulder blades squeezed when you lift the weights and when you lower them. Release your shoulder blades at the bottom of the movement.

How to Make It Harder: Use slightly heavier dumbbells.

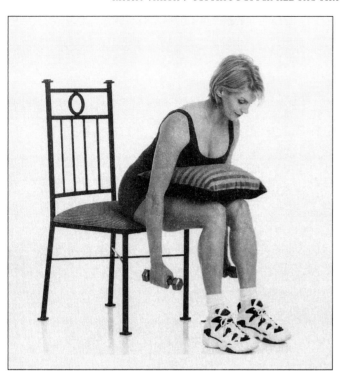

Seated
Back Flye
Position A

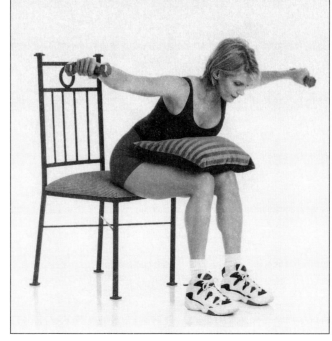

Seated
Back Flye
Position B

15. Standing Calf Raise

Works your calf muscles.

Starting Position: Stand on a sturdy platform facing the back of the chair, and rest both hands on the seat back for balance. Balance on the balls of your feet with your heels hanging off the edge of the platform.

The Exercise: Inhale, and slowly lower your heels until you feel a gentle stretch in your calf muscles. Exhale, and push up onto the balls of your feet, lifting your heels as high as you can. Pause at the top, inhale, and lower back down.

Technique Tips: As you lift up, keep equal weight across all ten toes. Counteract the tendency to roll your feet outward by pressing the big-toe side of your foot into the floor. To keep your balance, pull your abdominal muscles in and keep your buttocks tucked. Lift and lower at the same speed, taking two slow counts in each direction.

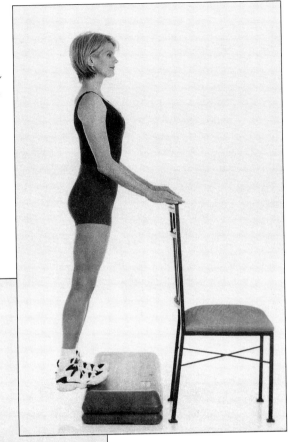

*Standing Calf Raise
Position A*

*Standing Calf Raise
Position B*

16. Toe Raise

Works your shin muscles.

Starting Position: Sit up straight in a chair with your feet flat on the floor. Place your right heel on the top of your left foot near your toes. Place your hands on the sides of the chair seat to help keep your back straight.

The Exercise: Exhale, and lift the front of your left foot off the floor, gently pressing down with your right foot to create resistance. Pause at the top, inhale, and lower back down.

Technique Tips: Lift your toes as high as you can off the floor, but maintain good posture, making sure not to slump. Resist on the way up *and* on the way down, pushing gently with your right foot.

How to Make It Harder: Add more pressure with your top foot, creating more resistance on the way up and down.

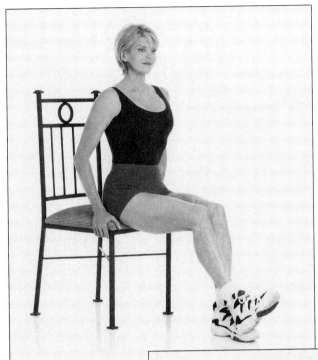

*Toe Raise
Position A*

*Toe Raise
Position B*

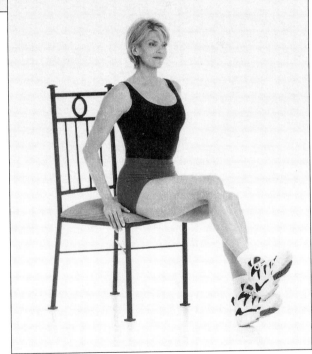

17. Rear Raise

Works the rear shoulder muscles and back of upper arm.

Starting Position: Use your light or medium dumbbells. Stand with your feet hip-width apart, knees slightly bent, abdominals tightened, and arms hanging by your sides. Hold a dumbbell in each hand, palms facing in.

Technique Tips: As you lift your arms back, try not to lean forward. Keep your body upright. Don't let your arms flare out to the sides; lift them directly behind you.

How to Make It Harder: Use your medium to heavy dumbbells.

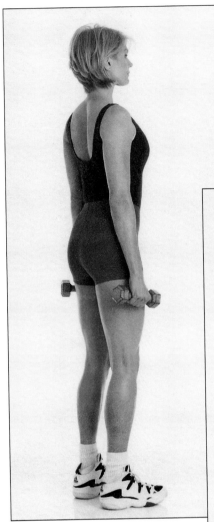

Rear Raise
Position A

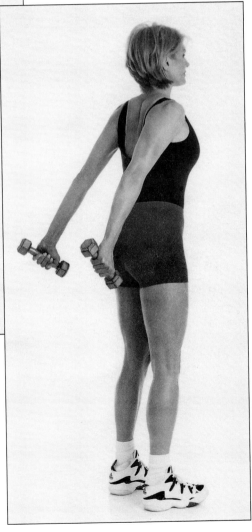

Rear Raise
Position B

18. Front Raise

Works the front shoulder muscles.

Starting Position: Use your light or medium dumbbells. Stand with your feet hip-width apart, knees slightly bent, abdominals tightened, and arms hanging by your sides. Hold a dumbbell in each hand, palms facing in.

The Exercise: Exhale, and slowly raise your arms in front of you until the dumbbells are slightly higher than your shoulders. Pause, inhale, and lower back down.

Technique Tips: Keep your elbows slightly bent, and don't allow your arms to lift higher than your shoulders. Keep your palms facing in the whole time. Try not to lean back as you lift, and don't swing the weights.

How to Make It Harder: Use your medium to heavy dumbbells.

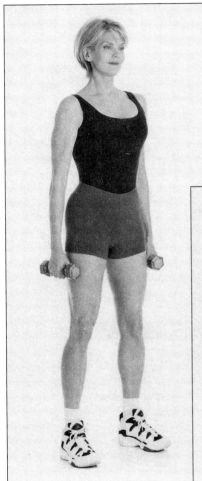

Front Raise
Position A

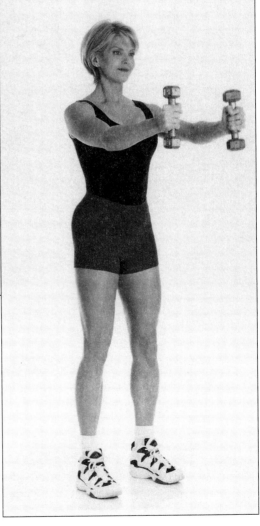

Front Raise
Position B

19. Backward Lunge

Works your buttocks plus back and front of thighs.

Starting Position: Stand up straight with your abdominals tightened, arms hanging by your sides, and feet slightly apart.

The Exercise: Inhale, and take a large step back with your right leg, bringing your hands to your hips. Bend both knees so your left knee is directly over your left ankle and your right knee points to the floor with your heel lifted. Your left thigh should be parallel to the floor. Exhale, and push off your right toes back to starting position. Alternate legs, doing the recommended number of repetitions for each leg.

Technique Tips: Throughout each repetition, keep slightly more weight on your front leg. If you have trouble balancing, place a chair at your side and grasp it lightly with one hand.

How to Make It Harder: Hold a medium to heavy dumbbell in each hand.

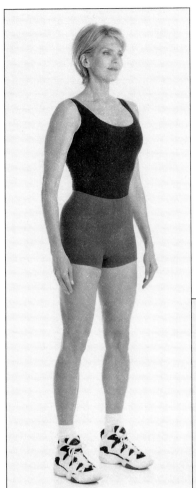

Backward Lunge
Position A

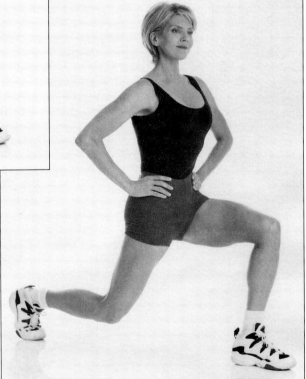

Backward Lunge
Position B

20. Back Extension with a Twist

Works your lower back muscles.

Starting Position: As in the Back Extension, lie on your stomach with your feet down, forehead resting on your hands, and elbows out to the sides.

The Exercise: This is a four-count movement: 1) Exhale, and lift your chest off the floor. 2) Twist your torso to the left until your right elbow touches the floor and your left elbow points diagonally toward the ceiling. 3) Return to center. 4) Inhale, and lower back down. Alternate sides until you've completed the recommended number of repetitions for *each* side.

Technique Tips: Let your lower back muscles do all the work. As you twist from your torso, don't rotate your neck; just let your head go along for the ride naturally. Don't let your feet lift off the ground.

How to Make It Harder: Repeat all of the repetitions on one side, then repeat the same number of repetitions on the other side. Do not alternate sides after each repetition.

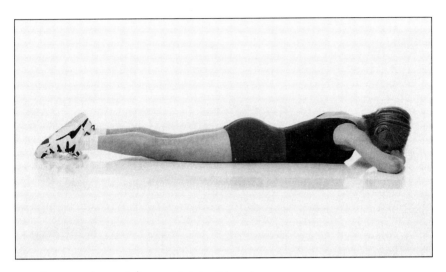

Back Extension with a Twist Position A

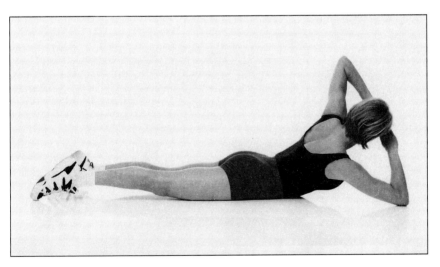

Back Extension with a Twist Position B

BREAKING STRENGTH PLATEAUS

Just as you occasionally hit plateaus in aerobics training, you will also get to that place where you feel you can't go any higher in your strength training. Which is why I'm going to give you an effective periodization program that you can do once you reach the "exercising regularly" level.

In this program, each phase will last two weeks, for a total of six weeks.

WEEKS 1 AND 2: This is the BUILDUP part of your cycle.

Begin by doing each exercise at a level where you reach moderate fatigue after eight to twelve reps. If you still haven't reached moderate fatigue after twelve reps, you'll need to increase the amount of weight a bit.

WEEKS 3 AND 4: This is the peak of your cycle.

During these weeks, increase the intensity of each exercise until you fatigue at only eight reps. Again, if you don't by eight, add some weight.

Also, don't rest between exercises. Just keep moving from exercise to exercise—but do each exercise slowly. It should take you about two seconds for the lift or effort part of each exercise, then about two seconds for the release part of each. If you go too fast, you'll use your momentum to move the weights and your muscles won't work as hard.

WEEKS 5 AND 6: The recovery phase.

Here, you decrease the intensity of each exercise until you reach fatigue at twenty reps. If fatigue doesn't come at twenty, add more weight. If it comes before twenty, decrease the weight.

Use this phase to refocus on form and technique. That way, when you go back to the harder—or heavier—phases, you'll probably be able to sustain that form.

Finally, make sure you stretch during each phase.

STRETCHING EXERCISES

If you're like most people, you may be tempted to skip the stretching part of your program after finishing your cardiovascular or strength workout. Please don't. If necessary, go back and review the previous section that discusses how vitally important stretching is to your health and fitness. Then choose to make it a priority, knowing that it's every bit as important as the other parts of your program.

Stretching Guidelines

1. Hold each stretch for ten to sixty seconds to the point of mild tension or tightness. Do not stretch until it hurts.
2. Relax and hold the stretch; don't bounce into it. This is called "static stretching," and it is the best and safest way to get the results you're after.
3. Stretch all of the major muscle groups in the body in order to achieve balance and symmetry. But you should pay particular attention to the areas in which you generally lack flexibility because of your lifestyle. Let's say you spend most of the day in a chair behind a desk, typing at a computer. You'll then need to concentrate especially on the chest and shoulder areas, the hip flexors and hamstrings, and the calf muscles.
4. Stretch when your muscles are warm. The best way to get them warm is through five minutes of some easy, rhythmic movement, including marching in place. Stretching cold muscles is more likely to cause strains or other injuries. Once the muscles are warm, then start slowly and listen to what your body tells you in the way of pain signals; don't stretch too far.
5. Maybe most important of all, try to relax as much as possible while stretching. If you begin to feel tension in other parts of the body than the one being stretched, ease off immediately and start again from the beginning . . . slowly, carefully.

The Stretches

These stretching exercises are listed in the order I'd like you to perform them. If you're just beginning, choose only the first five exercises, adding them (in order) as you progress.

THE STRETCHES

1. Hamstring (Back of the Thigh) and Calf

Technique Tips: Raise your right leg and rest your foot on a chair seat. With your right leg straight and left knee slightly bent, lean forward from your hips, not your waist, and pull your toes back toward you. You shouldn't have to tilt your upper body very far forward before you feel the stretch in the back of your leg and your calf muscles. Repeat with your left leg extended.

How to Make It Harder: Lean a little farther forward and pull your toes back toward you farther.

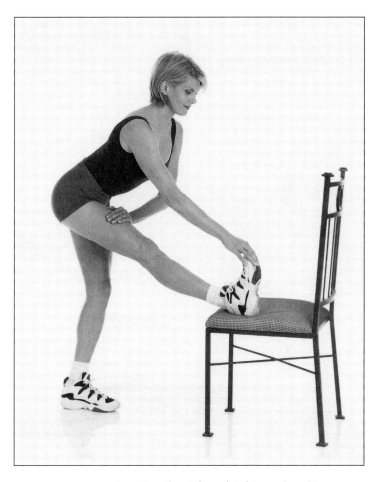

Hamstring (Back of the Thigh) and Calf

2. Quadriceps (Front of the Thigh), Hip Flexor, and Shin

Technique Tips: Place your left hand on a chair for balance, and grasp your right foot behind you with your right hand. Pull your heel gently toward your buttocks. Keep your knees together and hips facing forward. Repeat with the other leg.

How to Make It Harder: By squeezing your buttocks and tucking them under slightly, you'll feel an even better stretch in the front of your thigh and hip. If you point your toe, you'll feel more of a stretch in the shin.

3. Chest and Front of Shoulders

Technique Tips: Stand with your feet hip-width apart and knees slightly bent. Clasp your hands behind your back. Straighten your arms, then lift your hands and chest.

How to Make It Harder: Lift your arms a little higher behind your back, take a deep breath, and feel your chest expanding.

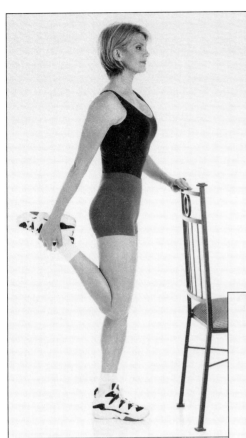

*Quadriceps
(Front of the
Thigh),
Hip Flexor,
and Shin*

*Chest and
Front of Shoulders*

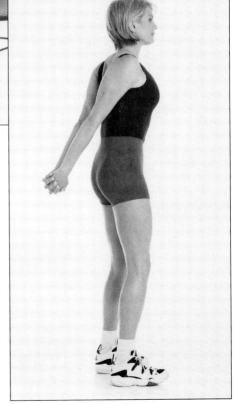

4. Neck and Upper Back

Technique Tips: Stand with your feet hip-width apart and knees slightly bent. Drop your head forward, until you feel the muscles in the back of your neck stretching. Slowly lift your neck back up. Now place your hands behind your back, and grab your right wrist with your left hand. Drop your head to your left shoulder, and at the same time pull down on your right arm, stretching your neck and upper back. Bring your back up, then repeat to the other side.

How to Make It Harder: This is a muscle group that should be stretched gently. As you hold the stretches, exhale and feel the release in the muscles that get tense from everyday activity.

5. Hips, Buttocks, and Abs

Technique Tips: Lying on your back, use your right hand to pull your left knee across your body and toward the ground on your right side. Keep your left shoulder flat on the ground with your arm outstretched. At first you may not be able to keep your shoulder flat on the floor, but you'll still get a good stretch in your abdominals. Repeat on the other side.

How to Make It Harder: By slightly altering where you place your bent leg, you'll feel the stretch in different parts of your hips and buttocks. Try moving your knee toward your head, then away from it.

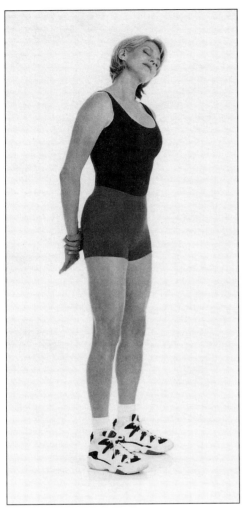

Neck and
Upper Back

Hips, Buttocks,
and Abs

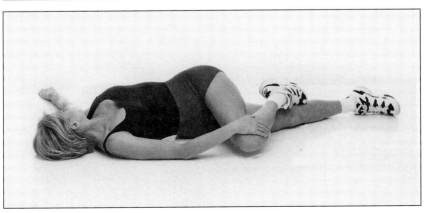

6. Inner Thigh

Technique Tips: Sit on the floor and bring the soles of your feet together. Now bring your feet in as close to your buttocks as you comfortably can. Use your elbows to push your knees toward the floor. You should feel the stretch on the inside of your thighs.

How to Make It Harder: Lean forward from your hips. Try not to round your back as you push your knees a little farther toward the floor.

7. Shoulders

Technique Tips: Stand with your knees slightly bent, and raise your right arm in front of you to shoulder height. Place your right hand on your left shoulder. Grasp your right arm with your left hand, and pull your right arm across the body. Repeat with your left arm.

How to Make It Harder: By moving your shoulder up toward your ear and then down as far as you can, you'll feel the stretch a little deeper in your shoulder and upper arm.

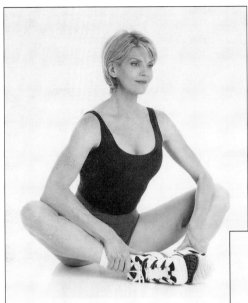

Inner Thigh

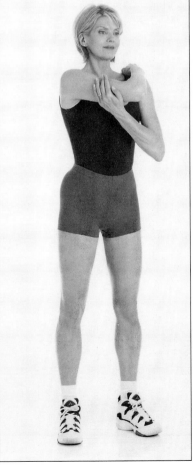

Shoulders

8. Back

Technique Tips: Kneel on all fours with your hands and knees spread evenly and your neck relaxed. Tighten your abdominals, drop your head, and round your back up like a cat would. Hold, then return to starting position.

How to Make It Harder: By tightening your abdominal muscles—as if you're pulling your navel to the ceiling—you'll allow your back muscles to really relax and lengthen. Open up your shoulder blades for more stretch in your upper back.

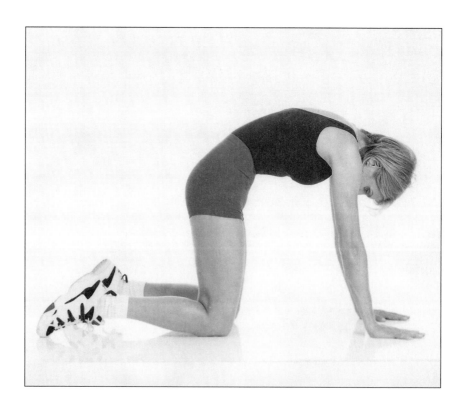

MAKING YOUR EXERCISE PLAN FIT INTO YOUR LIFE

Remember not to fall into the trap of thinking that your workout program has to be completed every day in one continuous segment. All the research indicates that you get the same health benefits by doing, say, three ten-minute bouts of exercise as you would from doing a single thirty-minute workout. So if you're short on time some days, go right ahead and break up your routine in manageable, bite-size pieces.

You can combine your three exercise categories in any order that feels comfortable and fits your lifestyle. For instance, you may like to get up early and do your strength training and stretching before work. Then maybe afterward you can meet a friend and take a walk, or go to the gym for an aerobics class. Or you may prefer to start your day with either a ride on your stationary bike or a walk, warming you up for your strength workout and stretching.

Most important, remember that the time you spend doing recreational activities with family and friends counts just as much as those dedicated workouts. Any activity, even vigorous housecleaning or gardening, burns calories and helps you to stay (or get) fit. If you find it's easier to "play" than to "exercise," by all means, choose activities that are more recreational.

If you're going to succeed at your workout program, you'll have to choose exercises that fit your tastes and temperament. So be creative in finding ways to make them a part of your life.

And if you fall off your plan for any reason, don't lose heart, believing that the game is over. Just get back with the plan immediately. Start where you can and progress to where you left off. You're the one in charge. You're the one who can make the plan successful. Only you. Only you can improve your health, your fitness level, your life in general.

Only you can make the kinds of choices that will take you to a future of health, happiness, and abundance.

Conclusion

What you've learned in this book will never fail you, whether in times of crisis or in times of joy. In almost any situation, you can apply the principles I've described. Once you start practicing them—and incorporate them into the fabric of your life—they will become second nature and serve you well. My sincerest hope is that you'll always believe in your power to change, and that you'll never forget the Power of Choice.

But please, be patient. Getting better all the time is an ongoing process. Life isn't easy, nor is it perfect. But, of course, people aren't perfect either. All of us have to deal constantly with ups and downs as we ride life's roller coaster.

As with amusement park roller coasters, we have a choice: enjoy the ride, or close our eyes in fear. I prefer to enjoy it, or at least to stay in the moment—applying the principles I outlined in this book. Utilizing the Keys to Success, adopting a healthy and nutritious eating plan, and exercising regularly has made my ride so much easier and infinitely more enjoyable. I know it can do the same for you, too. Gone will be that white-knuckle gripping to the sides of the roller coaster.

You have the power to change—to look on the bright side rather than the dark side, to embrace success rather than failure. It's time to assume control of your life, to brainstorm solutions to your problems rather than throw up your hands in despair, and to take action steps necessary to achieve your goals rather than staying stuck in the mud of hopelessness.

By committing yourself to healthy, nutritious eating—an integral part of my own success—you'll stop thinking of food as the enemy. And you'll no longer have to struggle with "dieting."

And remember that regular exercise is essential for both peace of mind and optimal health. It's never too late to start an exercise regimen that works for you, and that you can work into your life. If you do, I promise that you'll experience breakthroughs in countless other areas of your life.

I have every confidence that, with commitment, positive changes will occur in your life in ways you could never have imagined. Remember, life is a process—and so is Getting Better All the Time.

Please let me know how you're doing, I'd love to hear from you. Include a self-addressed, stamped envelope and I'll personally answer your letters.

Kathy Smith Lifestyles
P.O. Box 491433
Los Angeles, CA 90049

REFERENCES

1. S. A. Westphal, M. C. Gannon, and F. Q. Nuttall. Metabolic response to glucose ingested with various amounts of protein, *Am J. Clin Nutr.* 52 (1990): 267–272.

2. E. N. Whitney and S. R. Rolfes. *Understanding Nutrition. 6th Ed.* West Publishing Company, 1993. Pg. 109.

3. Gail Butterfield. Amino Acids and High Protein Diets. *Perspectives in Exercise Science and Sports Medicine, Custom Edition for Santa Monica College.* Ed Lamb/Grisolfi. Brown and Benchmark Publishers, 1993. Pgs. 108–110.

4. Melvin H. Williams. *Nutrition and Fitness for Sport.* Wm. C. Brown Publishers, 1992. Pgs. 127–8.

5. Edward N. Siguel and Robert H. Lerman. Role of essential fatty acids: danger in the US Department of Agriculture dietary recommendations ("pyramid") and in low fat diets. *Am J. Clin Nutr.* 1994: 60:973.

6. William D. McArdle, Frank J. Katch, and Victor L. Katch. *Essentials of Exercise Physiology.* Lon and Febiger, 1994. Pgs. 174–175.

7. Jacqueline R. Berning and Suzanne Nelson Steen. *Sports Nutrition for the 90's.* Aspen Publishers, Inc., 1991. Pg. 180.

8. Ulf Smith. Carbohydrates, fat and insulin action. *Am J. Clin Nutr.* 1994:59(supp): 686S–98.

9. F. Xavier Pi Sunyer. Health Implications of Obesity. *Am J. Clin Nutr.* 1991: 53: 1595S–1603S.

10. F. Xavier Pi Sunyer. Exercise in the Treatment of Obesity. *Obesity and Weight Control,* ed. Frankel and Yang. Aspen Publishers, Inc., 1988. Pgs. 251–252.

11. John T. Devlin. Effects of Exercise on Insulin Sensitivity in Humans. *Diabetes Care* 1992: 15 (S4): 1690–1693.

12. C. Bouchard, J. P. Despres, P. Mauriege. Genetic and nongenetic determinants of regional fat distribution. *Endocr Rev.* 1993: 14:72–93.

13. B. Y. Modugno. Insulin Resistance: A New Paradigm for Medical Nutrition Therapy and Nutrition Education. *SCAN Pulse.* Vol 14, No 4. F: 1995. Pgs. 1–4.

14. C. Wayne Calloway. Biologic Adaptations to Starvation and Semistarvation. *Obesity and Weight Control,* ed. Frankel and Yang. Aspen Publishers, Inc., 1988. Pgs. 105–106.

15. Gerald M. Reaven. Role of insulin resistance in human disease. *Diabetes* 37: 1495–607. 1988.

16. *Eating Disorders Review.* Vol 6, No 3, May/June 1995. Pgs. 1–4.

17. Bulow, J. Lipid mobilization and utilization. *Med Sports Sci.* 1988: 27: 140–163.

18. Ellen Coleman. Carbohydrates: The Master Fuel. *Sports Nutrition for the 90's.* ed. Berning and Nelson Steen. Aspen Publishers, Inc., 1991. Pgs. 50–51.

19. Paul B. Raven and Judy R. Wilson. Exercise for the Elderly. *Sports Medicine Digest.* Vol 10, No 6. June 1988. Pgs. 1–2.

20. National Restaurant Association Survey, 1993.

21. Douglas S. Brooks. *Program Design for Personal Trainers—Bridging Theory into Application.* Moves International Publishing, 1997.

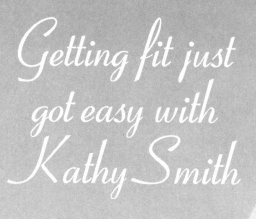

Getting fit just got easy with Kathy Smith

Two **NEW** Videos from America's Leading Fitness Expert™ take a fun, easy approach to exercise

- Two simple workouts based on everyday muscle group movements

- Tone and tighten lower body

- Train your body to burn fat hours after the exercise

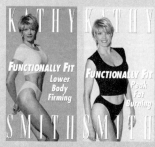

Now available wherever videos are sold

©1997 BodyVision All Rights Reserved. Distributed by WarnerVision Entertainment, Inc. A Warner Music Group Company

STAY ON TRACK WITH KATHY SMITH'S
WALKFIT™ AUDIO WORKOUT SERIES

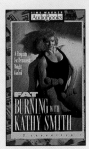

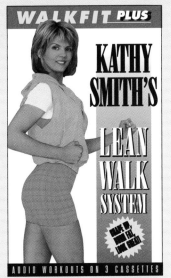

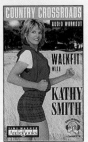

**FATBURNING WITH
KATHY SMITH**
1-57042-030-0
$15.00 (In Canada: $18.00)
Two cassettes,
2 hrs., 30-minutes

**KATHY SMITH: COUNTRY
CROSSROADS**
1-57042-370-9
$9.98 (In Canada: $11.98)
One cassette,
two 30-minute workouts

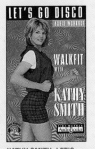

KATHY SMITH'S WALKFIT PLUS: Lean Walk System
1-57042-590-6/$19.98 (In Canada: $23.98)
Three cassettes, 3 hours

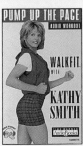

**KATHY SMITH: LET'S
GO DISCO**
1-57042-477-2
$9.98 (In Canada: $11.98)
One cassette,
two 30-minute workouts

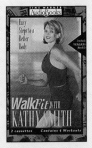

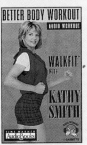

**KATHY SMITH: PUMP UP
THE PACE**
1-57042-476-4
$9.98 (In Canada: $11.98)
One cassette,
two 30-minute workouts

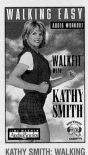

WALKFIT WITH KATHY SMITH
1-57042-020-3
$15.00 (In Canada: $18.00)
Two cassettes, three workouts

**WALKFIT WITH KATHY
SMITH: Better Body Workout**
1-57042-321-0
$9.98 (In Canada: $11.98)
One cassette, three workouts

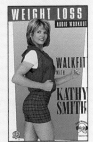

**KATHY SMITH: WALKING
EASY**
1-57042-466-7
$9.98 (In Canada: $11.98)
One cassette,
two 30-minute workouts

**Look for Kathy Smith's Fitness Walker,
high performance footwear
with a soft, cushioned
feel. Available at better
athletic shoe
stores.**

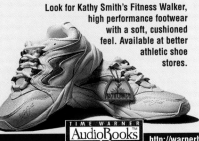

**WALKFIT WITH KATHY
SMITH: Weight Loss
Workout**
1-57042-324-5
$9.95 (In Canada: $11.95)
One cassette,
two 30-minute workouts

AudioBooks™ http://warnerbooks.com

©1997 WARNER BOOKS, INC.   A TIME WARNER COMPANY   THE TIME WARNER AUDIOBOOK NAME AND LOGO ARE REGISTERED TRADEMARKS OF WARNER BOOKS, INC.

If You Enjoyed *KATHY SMITH'S GETTING BETTER ALL THE TIME*, You'll Love Her Other Guides to a Healthy Body

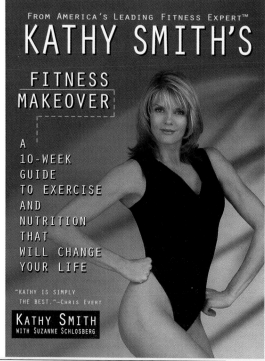

FROM AMERICA'S LEADING FITNESS EXPERT™

KATHY SMITH'S

FITNESS MAKEOVER

A 10-WEEK GUIDE TO EXERCISE AND NUTRITION THAT WILL CHANGE YOUR LIFE

"KATHY IS SIMPLY THE BEST."—CHRIS EVERT

KATHY SMITH
WITH SUZANNE SCHLOSBERG

KATHY SMITH'S FITNESS MAKEOVER: *A 10-Week Guide to Exercise and Nutrition That Will Change Your Life*
0-446-67049-9
$14.99
(In Canada: $18.99)
Trade paperback

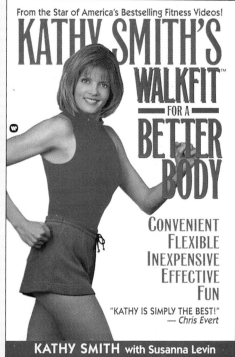

From the Star of America's Bestselling Fitness Videos!

KATHY SMITH'S WALKFIT™ FOR A BETTER BODY

CONVENIENT
FLEXIBLE
INEXPENSIVE
EFFECTIVE
FUN

"KATHY IS SIMPLY THE BEST!"
— Chris Evert

KATHY SMITH with Susanna Levin

KATHY SMITH'S WALKFIT™ FOR A BETTER BODY
0-446-67048-0
$8.99
(In Canada: $11.99)
Trade paperback

WARNER BOOKS

http://warnerbooks.com

©1997 WARNER BOOKS, INC.   A TIME WARNER COMPANY